I love how David Herzog explains the ancient mystery of how people used to live longer. It is supernaturally available today!

—SID ROTH
HOST, *IT's SUPERNATURAL!*

David Herzog has written an excellent book on not only how to look and feel your glowing best but also how to get off the sidelines and into the mainstream of your destiny. Many people cannot fulfill their purpose because of ill health, low energy, or mental fog. If that's you, *Jump Start!* is your practical guide to a new life. Do you need to lose weight? Heal your body? Turn back a few years? David points you in the right direction. Detoxing is a key to experience super natural health along with eating high-energy foods. When you remove toxins and feed your body super nutrition, your health will improve dramatically. I've seen this firsthand over and over again. This can happen for you. As David says, "An unhealthy body is suddenly changed into a healthy body." If you want super natural health, don't wait another minute to jump-start your journey to life.

—CHERIE CALBOM, MS, CN
AUTHOR, *THE BIG BOOK OF JUICES AND GREEN SMOOTHIES*
AND *THE JUICE LADY's LIVING FOODS REVOLUTION*

Today it seems that people of all ages are interested if not desperate to look and feel their best. Health information comes from many sources, providing conflicting information that leaves people confused and even hopeless. *Jump Start!* by David Herzog is a breath of fresh air providing the reader with a road map to achieving abundant health and life. With topics ranging from fitness and cleansing to improving your appearance and even strategies to reverse the aging process, *Jump Start!* will impart health knowledge into your life that can make a major impact. The principles taught by David Herzog are unlocking the health potential of people all over the world, and now it's your turn to experience a breakthrough in your own health and wellness. Your health is the greatest asset you have. Make the most of this life by treating your body like the temple it was created to be. Read *Jump Start!* today and begin living life to the fullest.

—JORDAN RUBIN
NEW YORK TIMES BEST-SELLING AUTHOR
OF *THE MAKER'S DIET*
FOUNDER, GARDEN OF LIFE AND BEYOND ORGANIC

I am happy to say I was one of the voices who encouraged David to do this project. While working with him in various conferences and dining in his home, I noticed that this dynamic man was very intentional about how he lived, what he ate, and the supplements he took—some of which are his own creation. As he, his wife, and children are vibrant and beautiful people, I asked about his philosophy of health. Within ten minutes he gave me an easy-to-understand yet powerful integrated strategy to maximize not only health but also physical and mental stamina while sculpting physical appearance. I wanted to see this in print—and am delighted he has done such a brilliant job. King Solomon referred to wise sayings as "apples of gold in settings of silver." This information is as priceless as it is sweet to read. *Bon appétit.*

—DR. LANCE WALLNAU
FOUNDER, LANCE LEARNING GROUP
DALLAS, TEXAS

David Herzog

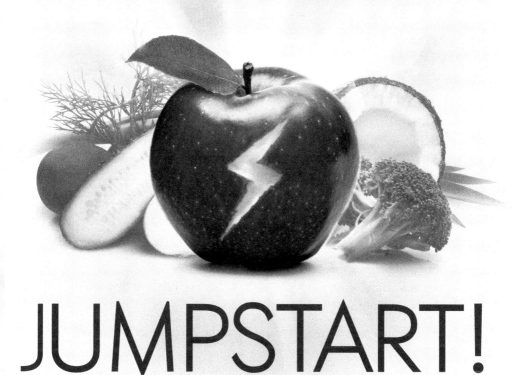

JUMPSTART!

SILOAM

Library of Congress Cataloging-in-Publication Data
Herzog, David.
   [Natural to supernatural health]
   Jump start! / David Herzog. -- First edition.
        pages cm
   Rev. ed. of: Natural to supernatural health. c2010.
   Includes bibliographical references.
   ISBN 978-1-62136-595-2 (trade paper) -- ISBN 978-1-62136-596-9
   (e-book)
   1. Mental healing. 2. Spiritual healing and spiritualism. 3. Health.
   4. Weight loss. I. Title.
   RZ401.H47 2014
   615.8'51--dc23
                                    2013039181

Portions of this book were previously published as *Natural to
Super Natural Health*, copyright © 2010, by DHE Publishing, ISBN
978-0984523504.

14 15 16 17 18 — 9 8 7 6 5 4 3
Printed in the United States of America

This book is dedicated to the Creator of heaven and earth for leading me in the direction of supernatural health and giving me the courage, motivation, and inspiration to write and finish this book. I will spend the rest of my life exploring the depths of the Creator and His wonderful creation, sharing it with the world.

I also want to dedicate this book to by loving wife, Stephanie, who stood by me during the countless hours of work and study to finish this book.

Also, a big thank-you to Megan Allison and Dana Grgurich for helping me research many of the sources in this book.

CONTENTS

TRANSFORM YOUR BODY INTO A LEAN, MEAN, SUPER-ENERGIZED BEING

EVERYBODY WANTS TO look and feel their best! I know because I have talked with, counseled, and helped people around the world from every sphere of life—single mothers, heads of state, actors, entertainers, athletes, construction workers, business leaders, spiritual seekers, students, and people on every continent and every social sphere. Everyone wants the same thing: a thin, vibrant, energetic, youthful, radiating, clear-skinned, super-healthy, blissful, toned, and muscular body. They want to be so super-charged and to live stress free. Not only do they want a healthy, fabulous body, but they also want to know sheer joy and inner peace while living out their destiny and dreams instead of just existing. Imagine having all that and being connected to the highest power source of love and peace!

Does that sound like what you are looking for? Does it sometimes feel there are physical, mental, emotional, and spiritual blockages that keep you in a stagnant stage of just going through the motions? As if there were invisible barriers somehow stopping you from having the willpower to go from existing to thriving in every area of life? Does this constant cycle keep you feeling sluggish—and at times frustrated that your body is not getting any younger or thinner, no matter what you try? Does this affect your actions? In addition to shedding extra pounds and achieving optimal health, do you want to demonstrate the courage to achieve your greatest desires? That is not only possible, but thanks to the advanced knowledge you are about to read in this book, it is also easier to realize than ever before.

Jump Start! will take you from a natural to a super natural, super-energized state that will create a more attractive and charismatic countenance. With a healthier, leaner body you will enjoy a drastic change in appearance and youthfulness, a new mental outlook on life, and the kind of stress-free, carefree standard of living you have always sought.

From Natural to Super Natural

When you start to shed excess pounds and cleanse your body, eat living raw and organic foods, super-energize your body, look ten to twenty years younger, and change your outlook on life, something else happens. In addition to feeling different on a physical level, you will tap into another spiritual plane. When you go for a nature walk, you will suddenly experience a sense of sheer love, joy, energy, peace, and happiness flooding your entire being. Not only are raw, natural, and organic foods releasing high levels of nutrients and energy, but because your newly cleansed and energized body is unclogged and fully alive, you will become more aware of the invisible world around you. Feeling sheer bliss, you will become thankful for the beauty all around you. Removing years of undesired toxins and waste in your body changes you into a channel for receiving immense levels of energy, joy, and peace. Thankfulness for life effortlessly overtakes you.

The principles in this book will start to work for you immediately, so as you read each chapter, start applying the keys and lifestyle changes. Go ahead and get excited right now about the new life that is just around the corner!

From Death to Life!

Once you delve into this book and experience the sheer ecstasy of your new life, you will never want to go back! When you think back to how you used to feel and live, you will feel as if you came back from the dead.

Many people are utterly confused by the myriad of claims from so many nutritional supplements, health products, TV infomercials, and other advertisements claiming to be *the* solution for energy, skin beauty, and health. Ultimately this information overload leads to more frustration once you realize most were empty promises. However, once you get hold of the truth, understand health at its core, and live out your new lifestyle, you will never again be easily swayed by the latest fad. Nor will you run to the nearest pharmacy to experiment with the latest drugs, most of which include major side effects. You will have the confidence and evidence of a truly super natural and super-energized body, one that vibrates on a much higher frequency. The moment you walk into a room, people will notice something powerful emanating from the inside out. In addition to glowing skin and a radiating, healthy body, people will notice a transformed human being enjoying the highest possible state of health in mind, body, and spirit.

How This Book Will Change Your Life

There are many health books on the market. Some focus on raw organic foods and others on cleansing. Some focus on exercise, and others proclaim to contain the latest scientific breakthroughs in health, medicine, and antiaging methods. Still others will focus more on the spiritual side of the human experience and how this affects your health. After having researched, studied, and lived a healthy lifestyle most of my adult life, I have endeavored to encompass all relevant information in an easy-to-read book, with motivational matter to help you get started right away. I have come to the conclusion that the only way to jump-start your way to super natural health is to take a multipronged approach. You need to hit it all at once on all levels, while exploring the latest cutting-edge, life-changing discoveries in natural, raw, and organic health.

As you read this book, you will find practical and natural solutions to some of your greatest health needs:

- ► A weight loss cure that really works

- ► More stamina and energy

- ► A diet full of miracle raw organic super foods

- ► Quick, easy, and effective exercises

- ► Antiaging secrets

- ► Hormone balancing

- ► A whole life refocus for total success and connection to the highest power source

In coming chapters I will deal with such topics as the super natural foods that will heal your body, boost your immune system, slow the aging process, and cause you to lose weight. As a quick example, in chapter 2 I will discuss plants, which are a prime source of pure energy that you should eat daily. The more you eat plants in their rawest natural form, the quicker you will possess energy, health, and vitality. This is because edible plants are a powerhouse of energy. On the other hand, processed food (think most anything that comes in a box or from the freezer section at the grocery store) with low or negative raw energy throws off your entire body. Synthetic, refined, and processed foods deplete the body of energy and strength.

I will also review foods that help your body operate at maximum efficiency by helping it to cleanse itself and relieve the stress that plagues millions who rely on the standard Western diet, which is full of fat and calories. Other chapters will deal with your mental and emotional states, which is huge in changing anything in your life. You will discover how to feel younger and what things you can do to naturally reverse the aging process. I will cover some of the easiest and most effective weight-loss methods that are healthy for you. These will not only make you lose weight but also reset your metabolism. At the end I will guide you through a twenty-one-day jump start to a super natural health plan so that you can see how to apply the principles of this book into your everyday life and experience the real results for yourself.

Remember that you are reading this book not by chance, but guided by divine destiny. You will discover truths you never knew about before. Get ready for the change of a lifetime!

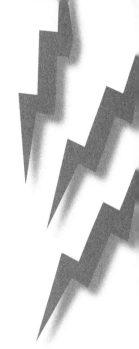

PART 1

GETTING JUMP-STARTED

Chapter 1

ARE YOU FIT AND FREE? IT'S TIME TO TAKE STOCK

*What you get by achieving your goals is
not as important as what you become
by achieving your goals.*[1]
—Naturalist Henry David Thoreau

IMAGINE YOURSELF IN a thin, vibrant, energetic, youthful, radiating, clear-skinned, super-healthy, blissful, toned, and muscular
body. Imagine living in a super-charged, healthy body, enjoying
stress-free days as you go throughout the week. Now go one step
further. What would it be like if you could enjoy more than a fabulous body and a carefree, stress-free life? What if you could also
wake up each morning with sheer joy and peace (inside and out)
because you are not only healthy but also living out your dreams
and destiny instead of just "getting by"? Does that sound and look
like what you desire? Not just another diet but an entire change to
your way of living life to its fullest? Yes, this is not only possible, but
it is also available. I believe you have picked up this book because
it is your destiny!

Does it sometimes feel that mysterious elements have conspired to obstruct your progress through life? These can be mental, physical, emotional, or spiritual blockages that keep you in a state of stagnation. While you wish it could be otherwise, simply going through the motions of survival leaves you feeling as if invisible barriers exist that prevent you from having the strength to break free. Yet it is possible to go from merely existing to thriving in every area of your life—starting with your health.

The results of the traditional Western lifestyle are often a constant, treadmill-like cycle that keeps you feeling sluggish and frustrated that your body is not getting any younger or thinner. No matter what you have tried in the past, this affects your motivation to get a jump start with your health and more. When you fail to realize a breakthrough in a vital area of your life, it also negatively affects your belief that you can pursue your other lifelong dreams. Weighed down, your mind starts to settle into "autopilot" mode. Instead of striving to improve, you settle for the ordinary instead of reaching out for a higher standard of living in every area.

Weighed Down

Have you ever thought that if you could just lose those extra pounds and be super healthy, you could also pursue your greatest desires in life? If you feel weighed down, you aren't alone. No matter where in the world you live, obesity represents a leading health problem, starting with the United States. Statistics released in 2013 by the Centers for Disease Control and Prevention (CDC) show that nearly 36 percent of adults ages twenty or older are obese, with a whopping 69 percent overweight. More than 18 percent of adolescents aged twelve to nineteen are obese, and a similar percentage of children ages six to eleven.[2]

What's worse, childhood obesity in America has more than doubled in children and tripled among adolescents over the past three decades. The CDC says among the immediate health effects of youth obesity are that youth are more likely to develop risk factors for cardiovascular disease, are more likely to have increased risk of diabetes in the future, and are at greater risk for bone and joint problems, sleep apnea, and social and psychological problems. Over the long term, they are more likely to be obese adults, which can lead to a host of health problems—heart diseases, type 2 diabetes, stroke, and cancer.[3]

Nor is this problem restricted to the United States. In 2013 the World Health Organization (WHO) reported that worldwide obesity had nearly doubled since 1980. In 2008 more than 1.4 billion adults aged twenty or older were overweight; of those more than 200 million men and nearly 300 million women were obese. This calculates to more than a third (35 percent) of adults being overweight and 11 percent having obesity. Nearly two-thirds of the world's population live in countries where being overweight kills more people than being underweight.[4] We are literally eating ourselves to death!

The CDC points out that healthy eating is associated with reduced risk for numerous diseases, including such leading causes of death as heart disease, cancer, stroke, and diabetes. I will address a healthy eating regimen and many other topics, but the most important thing to recognize as we start this journey is that losing weight and achieving optimal health is quite possible. In fact, you will find it easier than ever when you are equipped with the advanced knowledge that I will discuss in the coming pages. While most books focus on one subject—health, weight loss, antiaging, what foods to eat, or mental or emotional motivation—*Jump Start!* is different. It will touch all areas of your life and all at the same time. For example, you may go on a diet and lose weight, only to gain it all back because you fail to deal with other areas of life, such as emotional issues or mental blocks. This is because one area affects the other. When you push the "reset" button on all these areas at once, everything starts to change.

Personal Fulfillment

This book will deal with all those areas so that you not only get healthy and look better, you will keep it that way as you start to look younger and more vibrant, and feel more fulfilled. It is the synergy of all these human elements working together—along with a little help from above. I don't want you just thinner or healthier. I want to see you carefree and happy once again, like you were before life's burdens and responsibilities started to weigh you down.

Years ago, although fairly healthy and prone to take long walks and go to the gym regularly to work out, I still needed to lose some weight. I often felt sluggish and tired, as well as feeling that in some way I was not living life to the fullest. As I meditated on my situation and researched the subject of health and well-being, I realized that one area affects the others. Sluggishness in one area affects other areas and impedes your overall progress. I needed a total jump start. When I incorporated the secrets I learned into my life, everything started to change and brought benefits beyond what I could have imagined. People often said I looked ten to fifteen years younger. As a weight lifter, I already had a muscular build. However, after I shed about twenty pounds of excess hidden fat, I looked much different! Plus, when I "reset" my mind to where I would not allow negative thoughts to affect my will, I started accomplishing lifelong dreams. I would get stopped in airplanes, the grocery store, and malls as people—wondering if I was famous—asked for my autograph. This was before most people knew anything about me.

While I just wanted to be physically healthier, at the same time I found that my spiritual, psychological, and emotional health improved. Since the dramatic change in my life, people have approached me to ask if I am an actor, even naming different movies in which they thought I had starred. Others told me they sensed a natural high and energy just being around me and wanted to know my secret! CEOs of companies who bumped into me at a mall or in airports offered me jobs. Although they had no idea who I was, they assumed I could help their company. Creative ideas came effortlessly and started to generate huge success, causing major quantum leaps in my career.

Accomplish Your Destiny

When you allow your life to change physically, mentally, emotionally, and spiritually with no more blockages, you start to attract people and things that help accomplish your destiny. You will make connections you once thought impossible. Good things will gravitate your way! Take, for example, an old elementary school classmate named Dana, who now works full-time for my company. We had been in the same class as ten-year-olds. Many years later, after moving several times, I returned to my hometown, and Dana was still there. Her lack of geographical movement reflected the sluggishness of her life. Like millions of people, she was literally weighed down. She had tried numerous diets, only to fail and gain it all back. In addition, she suffered at times from a hard-to-explain anxiety, mood swings, and a general sluggishness. Happy and full of life one day, she found herself dreading the future the next.

Although generally happy, Dana recognized certain blockages had affected her life. After coming to work for me and starting on my program, everything started to shift. Dramatic physical changes improved her emotional outlook, which affected her family life…I could go on and on. First, she started losing the weight she always dreamed of losing, which thrilled her husband. Naturally, when this took place, she felt a new joy and excitement about life. This affected her work performance and eagerness to share her success with others. She is one happy camper and excited about each new day!

Once you delve into this book and experience the sheer ecstasy of life again, you will never want to go back! When you reflect on how you used to feel, look, and live, you will feel as if you came back from death to life. When you eat the right foods that nourish and replenish your body, you will cleanse your body and drop excess weight. All this affects you in dramatic ways. You will look ten to twenty years younger. When your outlook on life changes, impossibilities become possible. When things change on the physical plane, this new reality leads you to tap into another dimension. You can be taking a simple walk when suddenly waves of sheer joy, peace, energy, and happiness flood your entire being. Suddenly you feel more aware of the world around you. You start to experience sheer bliss just to be alive. Why? Because you are thankful for the beauty all around you—the beauty that, because of all the blockages surrounding your life, you could not appreciate before.

A Vibrant Life

I found it interesting that people who spend more time outdoors—even when completing the same exercises they would do indoors—experience greater weight loss, happier moods, and much lower levels of stress. I believe that the closer you get to something in its original state (such as creation), the more vibrantly you live on a higher level. Who doesn't like a barefoot day on the beach? Think about what areas of your life physically, emotionally, mentally, or spiritually could use a jump start. As you are thinking, take a look at this next section, so that you can accurately assess what areas in your life need that super natural jump start.

Where Are You?

However, you need to start where you are *right now*. You need to know where you are so that you know where you want to be. The simple checklists in this chapter will help you identify where you are and where you want to be in the next thirty days, as well as throughout the rest of your life. Be brutally honest in your evaluations, since this will provide the motivation to jump-start your quest for total health.

Answer each question in the checklists below by circling *Y* for yes or *N* for no. At the end of all sections, add up the total number of yeses and noes in the space provided. These questions will help you assess where you are in regard to foods and how you associate them with your thought patterns, emotional states, and exercise habits, as well as meditation or spiritual practices. When you answer the questions, base responses on your daily norms, not necessarily how you did today in regard to food or exercise. For example, if you just went to an all-you-can-eat buffet brimming with fatty foods, but you only do that a couple times a year, that would not be your norm. However, neither should you discount the volume of processed foods and unhealthy items like pizza, white bread, white pasta, and other starchy foods that may be part of your diet. One of the leading contributors to weight struggles is eating the wrong kinds of food.

Even though this book deals with the whole person, with each part intricately linked to the others, obesity is by far the number-one accelerator of sickness and aging. In addition to shortening your life span, it affects all the other areas of your life. Whether you need to lose as little as five pounds or as much as one hundred fifty pounds, once you start dropping this weight, this facilitates healing in every other organ of your body. It also affects the clarity of your mind, your emotional well-being, and your self-confidence. In turn, this affects your destiny and mind-set for accomplishing your life's purposes and dreams. Once you clearly assess your weaknesses and strengths, you will have a better idea of the elements of your situation that need the most emphasis.

Weight

1. I find it hard to lose weight, especially in my abdomen.   Y/N

2. I am addicted to desserts and sweets.   Y/N

3. I am at least fifteen pounds heavier
   than I was in my early twenties.   Y/N

4. I have trouble waking up in the morning.   Y/N

5. I often eat while watching television.   Y/N

6. No matter how much I exercise,
   I don't seem to lose the weight.   Y/N

7. I exercise less than one day a week.   Y/N

8. One or both of my parents are overweight.   Y/N

9. I often get less than eight hours sleep a night.   Y/N

10. I often go to bed past 11:00 p.m.   Y/N

Foods

1. I eat raw food every day.   Y/N

2. I crave fast foods and starchy foods like pizza.   Y/N

3. I eat more meats and carbs than veggies and fruit.   Y/N

4. I often eat late at night before going to bed.   Y/N

5. I mostly eat my vegetables cooked instead of raw.   Y/N

6. I drink less than 2 liters of water per day.   Y/N

7. I drink coffee every morning to get me going.   Y/N

8. I eat white bread, white pasta,
   and other white, starchy foods weekly.   Y/N

9. I am often an emotional eater.   Y/N

10. I tend to overeat when I am stressed.   Y/N

Thoughts/mind

1. I tend to gravitate to negative thoughts.   Y/N

2. I tend to worry more than I used to.   Y/N

3. I do not have the motivation that I used to.   Y/N

4. I often get distracted when working on a project.   Y/N

5. I tend to have a low self-esteem.   Y/N

6. I tend to get angry or offended easily.   Y/N

7. I have a hard time forgiving quickly.   Y/N

8. I believe I am fulfilling my purpose in life.   Y/N

9. I am daily making goals and working toward them.   Y/N

10. I tend to think of the past more than the future.   Y/N

Exercise

1. I exercise at least four times a week.   Y/N

2. I walk every day for at least forty-five minutes.   Y/N

3. I have a hard time getting motivated to exercise.   Y/N

4. I do not lift weights or use weight machines at a gym.   Y/N

5. I mostly exercise indoors.   Y/N

6. I feel great after I exercise.   Y/N

7. I don't feel that exercise is helping me when I do it.   Y/N

8. I do not find exercise enjoyable.   Y/N

9. I enjoy cardio more than weights.   Y/N

10. I enjoy doing sports more than exercising alone.   Y/N

Spirituality

1. I often have a quiet time meditating or praying. Y/N

2. I feel more spiritual when I am outdoors in nature. Y/N

3. Helping other people makes me feel spiritual. Y/N

4. I believe that there is a Creator but don't really pray. Y/N

5. I have a hard time being spiritual
   when my house is cluttered. Y/N

6. I would love to slow down and be more spiritual. Y/N

7. I am not part of a religious group
   but like to connect to God. Y/N

8. Helping others is my idea of being spiritual. Y/N

9. I don't feel that when I pray my prayers are being heard. Y/N

10. I am an atheist but would love to believe if I could. Y/N

Immune system

1. I often get sick at the same time every year. Y/N

2. I easily get sick when the seasons change. Y/N

3. I get less than eight hours of sleep a night. Y/N

4. I am often around electronic devices. Y/N

5. It takes me a long time to get better once sick. Y/N

6. I usually take drugs from the drugstore when I get sick. Y/N

7. I am tired most of the time. Y/N

8. I do not take supplements and vitamins. Y/N

9. I often smoke or drink alcohol. Y/N

10. I tend to get sick within a day or two of being angry. Y/N

What Are Your Results?

Total the number of yeses in each group and list them below:

Weight: ＿＿＿

Foods: ＿＿＿

Thoughts/Mind: ＿＿＿

Exercise: ＿＿＿

Spirituality: ＿＿＿

Immune System: ＿＿＿

If you have more yes answers in one particular group, then this is your area of most urgent weakness and where you need to focus.

Anytime you are weak in one area, it affects the others. Say, for example, that your emotional state is not good. This can affect your immune system and your weight. Or if you are overweight, this can affect your immune system and thoughts. You want to have total health in every area, starting with your weakest. If you answered yes two times in a particular group, this is a minor deficiency. If you marked between four and seven yeses, this is in the medium range. If you answered eight to ten in any one category, this signifies an urgent weakness. You need to jump-start improvements immediately. I will help you step by step.

Before concluding this chapter, though, I want to address two questions that often arise when I administer these checklists for various groups.

Why Thoughts and Emotions?

How you think, what you feel, and the quantities of food you consume are interconnected. Each affects the other. Certain eating habits are proven to cause weight gain and problems with your immune system. Some people associate certain foods with unpleasant experiences and create a mental block toward them. For example, some people have a disdain for green vegetables. Others have had a bad experience in the past with a diet or exercise regimen that did not work. When you learn to associate positive changes with healthy foods, the right thoughts, and the right exercise, things can quickly change for the better. Often it is a matter of breaking a negative pattern.

What If I Scored High in All Categories?

This just means that you need an overhaul. You are in the perfect place for this, or else you would not be reading this book. Even if you only need a little help, a little represents a lot. Often it is the last 10 percent of positive change that affects the other 90 percent of our existence. I believe it is no accident you are reading this book, which—if you follow it—will change your life. If you can visualize how you want to be in the next thirty days, you are already on your way. Keep seeing yourself the way you want to be.

When you begin this jump start into total health, something will happen to your mind. It will be uncluttered, and you will find emotional healing. This frees your spirit, allowing happiness and health to flow. I believe that there is more to us than meets the eye. People who allow their mind, body, emotions, and spirit to be healthy and recharged will experience the benefits of total health. My approach is to tackle all these areas instead of just one so you can see much greater, long-lasting breakthroughs. The results will be reflected not only in your physical health but also throughout your life.

Let's move on to the next section and discover how high-energy foods are key components in achieving super natural health.

•Chapter 2•

UNDERSTANDING NATURE'S ENERGY STORES

Tell me what you eat, and I shall tell you what you are.[1]
—Jean Anthelme Brillat-Savarin
Seventeenth-century French lawyer and politician

M ANY OF THE ancients lived off of the food that grew in the soil, untouched by modern-day food processing, genetically modified crops, and other so-called advances. Yet these "unenlightened" people seemed to possess super natural bodies and lifestyles. Contemporary food systems have deprived millions of people today of the euphoric feeling of healthy eating. In its place, mankind has created a multitude of new, previously unknown illnesses and diseases.

Remember, what you eat will determine your quality of life on earth, your mental and emotional state, and your spiritual well-being. Your body is a tool needing proper care and feeding to enable you to achieve maximum potential in every area of life. A correct diet that includes super foods gives you an edge over most other people. When you give your body these super foods, they propel

13

your mind, body, emotions, and spiritual life to new highs that you never could have achieved eating the standard Western, fat- and sugar-laden, carbohydrate-overloaded, meat-heavy diet.

When people fast for a season, they report having euphoric feelings, clear minds, and improved concentration. Sensing an enhanced connection with the spiritual world, they receive fresh and creative inspirations, ideas, and direction. This is because they temporarily cleanse their bodies from many of the harmful substances in modern foods. With nothing bad coming in, they detox during their fast and resurrect their spiritual senses. They don't deplete their energy digesting foods that overload the organs. Instead, they are connected to higher planes of thinking, feeling, and being. Once blockages are removed, their minds unclog. This allows them to think more creatively as their emotions come into balance and they feel much better physically—as if they can soar like an eagle during their fast.

Imagine having that same kind of feeling every day without fasting, yet eating in such a way that you are always on a natural "high" because of changing what you eat. With this new lifestyle you can go from a natural to a super natural being in a remarkably short time. You will find it much easier to achieve your lifelong goals and dreams because your mind, body, will, emotions, and spirit are congruently connected. All help you reach for your goals, with each enabling the other to progress.

Natural Foods and
Environments Restore Energy

Most people love to go camping, connect with nature, swim in the ocean, or go on nature hikes. You will notice that when you are on vacation in a natural setting, you feel more relaxed and under less stress. In this calmer environment you get fresh insights and inspiration. A major reason for this is the field of nature. Trees, rocks, and unspoiled forests carry a much higher energy frequency than metropolitan areas and downtown inner cities, where most everything is man-made and brimming with pollution. Most artists enjoy natural surroundings in the mountains or on the beach, where they can seemingly tap into a higher level of creativity. The closer you get to raw creation, the closer you draw to the Creator and the fresh, creative thoughts and abilities you would not otherwise experience.

Most people living in stressful city environments consume less-than-nutritious, "dead" foods and swim in the shark-infested waters of urban life. Operating in survival mode, they fight traffic morning and evening in the ill-named rush hour, hoping to arrive home at a reasonable time—only to watch toxic TV or Internet programming that increases stress and cortisone levels.

The foods you eat also carry certain various levels of energy. Even objects and people possess varying levels of energy. Let me explain. Energy is matter. Everything you see consisting of matter is made up of energy. Although more than a century has passed since physicist Albert Einstein first developed his special theory of relativity, $E = mc^2$ is still a fact today.

The idea that some foods have higher energy fields than others has been well documented. In 2008 the documentary *The Beautiful Truth* reported on the team of scientists that used specialized photography to analyze various foods. Organic foods contained a more vibrant and harmonious energy field than conventional foods, just as raw foods proved better than cooked and pasteurized foods.[2] Other researchers have photographed the energy levels of various objects, including fruit. In one photo a fresh, uncooked fruit looks like a supernova sun as it explodes with brilliant light. In the next photo the same fruit in cooked form emits almost no light. Plus, it looks somewhat deformed. Organic and raw foods have higher energy fields because their energy has not been destroyed or altered by unnatural processing or other means.

When you eat food that explodes with energy, you become

supercharged and full of energy as well. It is really true that you are what you eat. The higher the energy field of the foods you eat, the healthier you will be. Some foods are considered "dead" since they carry almost no energy while zapping you of health and vitality. The highest energy-rich, super foods are raw plant foods. They are the most perfect for human consumption. The reason: plants derive their energy directly from the sun. When you eat them, you ingest that energy directly into your system. Super foods cleanse and energize your body and rapidly exit your system.

The cleaner your body, the more you will radiate with good health. When you advance from a natural to a supernatural state, others will notice and be affected by what they observe.

Cooking food destroys most of the enzymes and nutrients; if that is the majority of your diet, you are obtaining much less nutrition from your food. Because they contain much lower nutrients, it often takes more cooked food to achieve a full feeling, which contributes to weight gain and increases the toxins you ingest. Your ideal detoxification goal is eating at least 80 percent raw food to start your journey to super natural health.

A toxic life and environment destroys your energy, joy, and outlook. With dulled senses and super natural abilities, you degenerate into a less vibrant creature than God created you to be. A toxic life causes you to live in a lower, survival mode instead of a creative, supercharged, "excited about life" state of mind. Once you change your food intake, dormant abilities resurface. Suddenly you will feel happy, positive, and fully charged—able to live your life to its fullest potential in every area as you call on your untapped genius!

Raw Plant Food = Super Natural

Raw plant foods are the ultimate source of pure energy. You should eat these pure, healing foods daily. The more you eat substances in their rawest, natural form, the quicker you will possess incredible energy, health, vitality, and strength on your way to a total transformation. Edible plants are a powerhouse of live, instantly absorbed energy fields. Since they receive energy directly from sunlight and fresh air, in turn you will ingest living, powerful energy fields. Consequently your energy vibrations will increase. On the other hand, when you eat processed food with low or negative raw energy, it throws off your system. Synthetic, refined, and processed foods deplete the body of energy, strength, and health. Slowly but surely this type of lifestyle eating robs you of health, joy, and freedom, spiraling your body toward death. Though the descent is slow, you will reach the grave at a younger age.

The idea is to try and consume as much raw food as possible. Most people can start by eating at least 50 percent raw foods and gradually increase to 80 percent raw plant foods and 20 percent cooked foods. Cooking destroys the enzymes in food that help to break down that food. The more enzymes you get throughout the day from raw foods, the faster they can flush toxins and junk out of your body. This continually cleanses, heals, and energizes you instead of clogging your system.

Different foods carry different levels of energy fields. The higher the food energy, the better it is for you. Anything that alters the food lowers the energy frequency, whether microwaving, canning, freezing, adding pesticides, or cooking. For example, frozen food destroys anywhere from 30 percent to 60 percent of the enzymes in the food. Yet it is still better and less damaging than cooked food. The bottom line: the more natural you go, the better. Everyone has to start somewhere, and knowing the different levels of natural to unnatural food really helps make the transition.

Energy Foods

High-energy food

Eating fresh, raw organic vegetables and organic, sun-ripened fresh fruit top the list of high-energy foods that will quickly take you from natural to super natural. The more raw green vegetables and raw fruit you eat the better, especially those that are organic and not tainted by pesticides.

Medium-energy food

Though not as high energy as raw plants and fruits, other foods that contain more energy than most cooked foods are things like some cooked vegetables; raw, organic goat milk and cheese; raw, organic nuts and seeds; and raw sprouted grains. These are considered medium-energy foods.

Lower-energy food

Some lower-energy foods that are still acceptable during a long-term transition to high-energy foods are free-range, organic eggs; organic wild fish (such as wild salmon, which is much higher in energy than beef or chicken and digests much quicker); raw cow's milk; and raw, cold-pressed oils. As you transition from dead foods to higher-energy foods, you will most likely be eating a mix of high-, middle-, and low-energy foods.

Neutral foods

There are some foods that are neutral, though not ideal for daily consumption as you transition toward your goal of replacing destructive foods with healthy ones. Examples: free-range, grass-fed, and organic meats; whole-grain products; and non-raw, organic cheeses (though something like raw goat cheese is superior).

Dead and destructive foods

If you hope to walk the path to total health, these are foods that you should stop eating right away. For starters, this includes pasteurized dairy products of any kind, including regular pasteurized milk, yogurt, and cheese (though raw is fine). The reason is that the pasteurization process destroys all the enzymes and nutrients in dairy products, leaving nothing but digestive and other complications. Other destructive foods, starting with the most detrimental, are nonorganic, farm-raised animal flesh; organic and/or grass-fed pork, shrimp, and lobster (all are bottom feeders); and nonorganic and non-free-roaming (hormone-infested) cow meat (beef), chicken, lamb, game, and farm-raised fish (wild fish is the best choice).

These dead foods are filled with hormones and steroids that stay in the meats and, consequently, enter your bloodstream. For example, pork is the worst because it literally clogs up your arteries more than any other meat. It also contains the highest amount of parasites and is not necessarily designed for human consumption. Doctors often tell people with clogged digestion to stop eating pork. Nonorganic and non-pasture beef, chicken, and most mainstream, nonorganic meats are so full of hormones and other chemicals that they slow you down and reverse the body's natural healing processes. (For example, organic beef from cattle that has been raised exclusively on grass has less saturated fat and more nutrients that grain-fed beef.) These also take the longest to digest and eliminate from your system. Any food that stays in your system for a long time tires you out the most. It also has the highest probability of causing sickness. (Remember the last time you had that huge, nonorganic late-night steak dinner? Chances are you soon felt pretty drowsy after the meal.)

Whatever food does not get digested quickly will stay in your colon, building up fecal matter. It also putrefies along the walls of your intestines, causing colon and other problems in the future.

When everything in your body starts to slow down, it blocks the absorption of nutrients, which causes many other problems over the long haul. While you don't have to be a strict vegetarian, if you focus on meat like wild fish while staying on high-energy foods with the occasional organic meats, you will fare much better than most people. Proceeding at your own pace, strive to eliminate most meats while adding more high-energy foods. Your goal is to eliminate destructive food from your diet as soon as possible.

Juicing and Blending

I call this the secret to tapping into the raw power of food. Fresh, raw organic vegetables and fruits that have just been juiced or blended are the most concentrated, edible, energy-filled nutrients that exist! When you use a juicer or blender, super natural liquid energy bypasses chewing and shoots nutrients and raw energy straight into your bloodstream. This provides a euphoric high—raw food in liquid form. Juicing and blending raw food smoothies not only tastes incredibly good, but it is also the fastest route of changing from natural to super natural eating. All you need to do is mix some fruit with the raw plants; the taste and sensation are out of this world. You are hydrating and oxygenating your cells every time you liquefy fresh, raw veggies and fruits.

What I like to do soon after waking up in the morning is to make a liquid, super-food drink. This is the first substance to hit my body for the day, causing a super natural energy burst before I eat anything else. I often like to throw in some spinach, kale, celery, and apple along with either water or coconut water for added flavor. In a few seconds you will have liquid, ready-to-consume energy! You are on your way to sensations of pure bliss! Once you see the major difference this makes in your health and mental outlook, you will wonder why you went on eating the way you did. (Just stick to this as a lifestyle, not a temporary diet. Going back to dead foods once you are on high super natural energy diets will often leave you feeling depressed.)

Blenders vs. Juicers

People use juicers because they feel they will get more nutrients into their diets this way. Juicers are different from blenders; they use an extractor to extract only the juice of fruits and vegetables while removing the pulp and fiber. The theory is that by removing the fiber, your body can easily absorb much higher levels of nutrients directly into the bloodstream. However, there is a potential problem with this. For example, if you are juicing sweet fruits and carrots, then their high-sugar content will cause a spike to your blood sugar. The fiber that would have otherwise balanced out the sugar has been removed. Nature intended that we consume the whole food. Juicing works best if you are using dark green, leafy vegetables. In this way you can maximize the nutrients you receive for your bloodstream, but without a spike in sugar.

Because juicing removes fiber—often the most nutritious part of a food—you can also become constipated if you do a lot of juicing and fail to get adequate fiber in your diet. As an example, the white skin of oranges is packed with phytonutrients, which you really need. When it comes to fruit, it is better to eat a raw, organic fruit than to juice it. Juice goes down quickly, is digested quickly, and absorbed into the bloodstream quickly. As a result, you become hungrier more quickly. Since smoothies contain fiber, you will feel full longer. And since high-fiber content takes longer to digest, you won't become hungry as quickly. Further, since juicing requires many fruits and vegetables, the juice—ounce for ounce—is *higher in calories and sugar* than a smoothie made in a blender.

Over the years I have used numerous blenders. The one that outlasts others (hands-down) is the Vita-Mix. Much larger than other blenders, it can handle the largest amount of food and is the sturdiest. It can even liquefy the pit of an avocado. The great thing about blending is that you get the entire fruit or vegetable, as if you chewed it. This way all the nutrients are in the food, especially the fiber. It is the ultimate tool to make quick, delicious meals. As I said earlier, raw smoothies made with your blender are very tasty. A juicer is much more time-consuming and takes much longer to clean.

It is easier to pack in more nutrients with a blender than by just eating a salad. You will also get it into your system faster, since the blender does the work of "chewing" the food into liquid form. This saves you time in eating, which can help you avoid thinking about relying on convenience or fast foods when pressed for time. To make a huge organic salad and eat it could easily take you an hour. But just throw such ingredients as spinach, kale, avocado, and an apple or two in your blender, and you can drink it quickly and be on your way. You will get all the same raw nutrients more quickly than by eating them, and much quicker absorption into your system! When blending, you are still getting the whole food as if you chewed it as nature intended.

If you have the time and want to get the most out of juicing and blending, then the best way is to juice your vegetables and pour the juice into a blender, adding fruits into the blender so that you keep the fiber content. Combining juicing with blending gives you the best of both worlds. As far as vegetables go, juicing is very beneficial. Many who are sick have used it to promote quick healing. Veggies that are blended usually take about two hours for absorption and digestion, but only thirty minutes when juiced. However, if you don't have much time and are just embarking on your jump-start trail, you still will get benefits from putting raw veggies and a little fruit into the blender, compared with not doing anything. Plus, your food will be much easier to absorb.

Why Organic?

Some people argue that it is too costly to buy organic. In reality, it is more costly *not to* eat organic. Consider the lower nutritional value of most foods and the sicknesses, diseases, and health care costs that stem from eating them. In addition, with most modern sicknesses, the majority of doctors don't focus on curing them but controlling the sickness with drugs that often have harmful side effects. In the long run, spending the extra money is worth it. Even in the short term, you will reap immediate benefits. Think of it as investing in your own health care so you don't have to be operated on or "experimented" with via pharmaceutical drugs at a later date.

Organic foods promote good health because they are in their raw, natural state. They are not sprayed with pesticides, chemicals, fungicides, and other harmful substances. Organically grown food also has much lower quantities of toxic trace minerals, such as lead, mercury, and aluminum. Plus, various studies have shown that organic food contains much more iron, potassium, magnesium, and calcium than conventional crops. Most studies show organic food has up to ten times the mineral content of conventional foods. You really get more nutrition for your money!

It is amazing how much fuller (faster) you will feel eating a smaller portion of raw organic food than processed. Before I changed my lifestyle, I remember going to get a hamburger at a fast-food place; I could eat a fistful of those burgers. The reason: my body was not getting the nutrients it needed, so it continued telling me that I was still hungry. In reality, that food is just being stored and contributing to weight gain. Such unnatural foods get stuck in your gut, confused as to where they should go in the body. On the other hand, I can eat an organic salad with lettuce, avocado, and other fresh vegetables, and one serving usually fills me up. Getting all the nutrients and healthy fats it needs, my body tells me that I am full.

Not only will you feel fuller, but also you will ingest far more nutrients. For example, smaller organic oranges contain 30 percent more vitamin C than the large conventionally grown ones. Other tests done showed that a serving of organic lettuce, spinach, carrots, potatoes, and cabbage provided the recommended daily intake of vitamin C, but the same veggies grown by conventional farming did not. Organically grown berries and corn had 58 percent more polyphenols—antioxidants that help prevent cardiovascular disease—and up to 52 percent more of vitamin C than conventional berries and corn.[3]

Easy In, Easy Out Foods

Foods that your body can digest quickly are the best—namely, more raw, organic food. Raw plants and raw fruits are the easiest to digest. They do not stay in your system but work to get in and get out as fast as possible.

Once you have started a cleansing regimen with a combination of colonics and other cleansing tools, it would be crazy to go back to a normal diet and get clogged up again. Let's say you are just starting to shift from an unhealthy, low-energy diet to a high-energy diet when you order a steak-and-potatoes type meal. Well, that dinner will spend eight to twelve hours in your stomach. As it takes the entire night to digest, it saps your body of vital energy needed to cleanse organs like your liver. While you sleep, your liver is being clogged up as it works overtime, trying to compensate during what should be a restful evening. You wake up feeling tired and groggy because your body did not really rest. It played catch up with all-night digestion.

On the other hand, if you ate a raw salad with that steak, as bad for you as the steak would be, just by adding that salad, the time in your stomach would be reduced to only four to five hours. This alone would greatly reduce your bloating, weight gain, and system clogging. Often, when you think you are craving meat, you are actually craving healthy fats, like avocado. Try making an avocado salad and notice how your meat cravings will drastically diminish, especially *in the evening*.

You see where I am going with this? Any changes you start to make with the goal of going between at least 50 percent raw food, on up to 80 percent, will make a dramatic impact on your life and health! Of course, the better meal would be wild salmon with the salad. That would digest much faster than the steak, particularly if you are just starting your plan. Imagine if you did not eat meat at night, since most weight gain stems from whatever you eat after 6:00 p.m. Imagine the energy you would have upon awaking, followed by a breakfast smoothie of raw organic vegetable and fruit juice. The more alkalized and raw the food you eat, the more it will prevent waste matter building up, which will keep you full of health, vitality, and energy!

That's why I am going to share with you several ways to cleanse your body of all the junk in the next chapter. As you cleanse your body, you will unleash all that extra energy you have been using maintaining a clogged system. With a more rested body, you can tap into the creative side of your brain and find fresh ideas. When you are weighed down by dead food, it clouds your thoughts, making it tougher to focus your thoughts. With a clear mind, you can act as a receiver of ideas, innovations, inventions, and projects that were there all along. However, you could not grasp them until you jumped from natural to super natural health.

Chapter 3

JUMP-START YOUR HEALTH
WITH A CLEANSE

*We are much better off taking a daily approach,
and being supportive, to the cleansing organs
that are designed to detoxify our bodies.*[1]
—Dr. David K. Hill,
author of *Nature's Living Energy*

To JUMP-START YOUR journey from natural to super natural health, the first step is cleansing. As your body cleanses itself of toxins—the impurities and other "stuff" that are part of many countries' food systems and environments—it will suddenly function at optimal, supercharged levels. This may sound like one of those "magic pill" infomercials that air in the wee hours of the morning, but this one is different: it is true! You will see yourself advance from natural to super natural health as you tap into infinite possibilities. The benefits encompass not just the physical but also mental, emotional, and spiritual.

You have likely heard the expression "What goes up must come down." Well, this is equally true: "What goes in must come out."

The problem is that much of what most people eat today does not all come out of their bodies very quickly. Instead, it stays inside far too long inside the intestines, rotting and causing complications. This is why I can promise that when you eat food that is alive and vibrant, organic, and raw, you will feel the same energy levels encompassed by these foods. You will feel internally cleaner, lighter, and less weighed down. This will affect your emotions, energy levels, and desire for the super natural. When you eat foods that have been robbed of nutrition and life, that death process affects your body. It is the same life spiral in reverse, which dampens your mind, will, and emotions.

When you are in natural settings, be that amid a mountain range or gazing out over the ocean, you feel more inclined to eat better and to exercise. You also become more spiritual and prone to pray, meditate, sing, and explore the spiritual world. This is because such blockages as tiredness, stress, and man-made surroundings no longer obstruct your life. In the same way, when your body takes in raw nutrients in their most natural form, these nutrients release a much higher energy. This leaves you feeling euphoric and helps you heal. When you eat man-made, processed food, you are ingesting food particles with broken-down atoms and sound waves—not to mention less nutritional qualities—which leaves you feeling less energized.

When you are often tired, sluggish, easily annoyed, or stressed, these are indicators that you are most likely blocked and clogged in several ways and not getting that direct energy high that you could. Healthy eating and living can be one pathway to release yourself into higher realms of health and the super natural. Through healthy eating and living, you can go from natural to super natural health!

Detox and Cleansing

As the seasons change, whether from hot to cold or cool to warm, many people get the flu or colds. This signals that your body is telling you it is time to detox and flush out the impurities. If you do this willingly, you don't have to experience the same "forced detox" that nature often brings upon us when we are overloaded. I often fast or cleanse my body at the start of a new season and notice that I seldom catch whatever new virus or flu is coming around. This is because healing can occur during detox. Often, as you start to cleanse your body, your emotional, mental, and spiritual outlook will also experience a detox. All that is negative will start to flush out or come to the surface.

Most people in the Western world have parasites known as Candida. Their intestines are bloated because of undigested meats still lying in the gut and stomach lining, putrefying the entire system. The list of ailments goes on. The entire body needs a full cleansing to launch the journey toward super natural health, including the liver, gallbladder, colon, and skin. As you detox, you will start to notice a radical transformation. You will be filled with youthful vigor and energy and will appear younger. Not only will your skin and complexion glow, but you will also experience weight loss, thickened hair, and an overall light feeling that you may have not felt since childhood. Others will notice your positive look—and outlook.

Once you cleanse the toxins and blockages from your system, you will radiate like never before. Nothing will slow or stop you by blocking your energy paths. You will start to tap into super energy and even super natural realms that you could not access when weighed down by obstructions. With everything unclogged, your mind will be much clearer and your emotions much more balanced. A clean body radiates life, light, and joy and is attractive to other people. This new state of cleansing and health will naturally draw others to you.

Once it is clean, your body will go from survival and decay to rebuilding itself. Freed from being overburdened with various toxins, your body can devote its energy to working on healing and rejuvenation. In this cleansing process, many people report different sicknesses, such as certain allergies and other ailments such as migraines, joint pain, sinus congestion, and skin problems just vanish. When I started to cleanse, I noticed allergies that would come every year from the pollen in the air would start to diminish or vanish altogether as my body was now able to resist and fight them. Also, I travel worldwide extensively, and I noticed my energy levels were much higher and I was able to bounce back quickly after such long grueling trips. My skin also started to clear up, and even my thoughts were clearer, as it seems to clear up "mental sluggishness" when your body is clean and functioning as it should. One of the best, most thorough ways to start a major cleansing process is colon hydrotherapy.

Colon hydrotherapy

This accelerates the detox process and will add years to your life. By enabling you to quickly detox without hindering your daily life, it helps avoid dealing with extreme symptoms that can arise during a slow cleansing process. It is simple, painless, and discreet. Just find a licensed colon therapist; in the day and age in which we live, colonics are vital to your health to thoroughly eliminate impacted fecal matter and toxins. The methods used in this process have been around for thousands of years. A series (anywhere from six to twelve) of colonics once or twice a year is a good start.

The goal is to empty out your bladder, colon, liver, and intestines from years of backed-up fecal matter and decay—usually meats—rotting in your body from undigested food. This will allow your lymph system to drain. The other important thing is that you will be flushing out encrusted mucus, which poisons your system and feeds parasites. Usually after a few colonics, the liver starts to cleanse, propelling you on your way to super natural health. You can expect to see a dramatic flattening of your stomach; many people lose between five and twenty pounds just from a series of colonics! Also, you will drastically reduce bloating, gas, food cravings, and constipation—not to mention improved digestion, increased energy and mental clarity, a better absorption of nutrients, and overall improvement in your health.

Wrote the New York–based editor of *Health* magazine after undergoing a colonic: "Afterward, Brigit escorted me to a private bathroom—some people have to go after, some don't—where a trip to the scale showed that I was 2.4 pounds lighter! But even better than the instant deficit on the scale was how I felt, both physically and mentally. I walked in feeling tired, sluggish, bloated. I walked out feeling totally rejuvenated, ready to run a marathon, and with a super-flat tummy to boot. I felt even better the next day and raved about my clean colon to anyone and everyone who would listen."[2]

Probiotics

During your series of colonics you should take probiotics to ensure healthy digestive conditions and a healthy bacterial flora as you rid yourself of the "bad stuff." These supplements will put friendly bacteria into your system that will trigger your metabolism, improve digestion, and help with the cleansing. I recommend taking them on an empty stomach right after your colonic and during the following three days.

During your colonic series you will also want to alkalinize your body with lots of greens and green-leafy vegetable juices. With colonics, chlorophyll and chlorella help to speed up the detox process by pulling out harmful toxins from the body, such as heavy metals, mercury, and foreign chemicals. To re-mineralize your body, you can buy encapsulated organic supplements, such as blue-green algae, chlorella, and organic spirulina.

Liver detox

One of your primary objectives is to detoxify the liver. Once that happens, all the other organs follow. Most people have a clogged or sluggish liver. This can lead to things such as your metabolism slowing down as fat stores increase, digestion slowing down, appetites increasing, and food cravings increasing. When this occurs, your body's immune system and liver get overloaded, causing symptoms and diseases over time. The liver will detoxify even more quickly when fasting on juice or fresh spring water, as it will be less overloaded with excess toxins.

A consistent diet of cooked animal foods and fried foods without the balance of raw foods is difficult for the body to metabolize. By reducing or eliminating animal and fried foods during the cleansing process, you will help your body with its goal of flushing out old waste matter so you can nourish it with super foods. When you cleanse your liver, because it is no longer overtaxed, every organ in your body starts to function more efficiently. As a result, you will experience more energetic (and euphoric) feelings and increased metabolism, you will feel less compelled to overeat, and you will have an enhanced sense of well-being. Only do a liver cleanse after you have done a series of colonics and your body has started to rebuild.

An unhealthy body will suddenly become changed into a new healthy body through detox. Eating living foods will help with mental clarity and a positive outlook. While colonics will start to cleanse your liver, it is helpful to do a separate liver cleanse after a series of colonics.

There are different ways to do a liver cleanse. A seven-day juice cleanse with specific juice recipes for the liver is one; another option is to take liver cleanse supplements, which are typically a five-day regimen. You may also choose to eat liver-supporting foods that will help your liver naturally detoxify, such as garlic, grapefruit, green vegetables, avocados, walnuts, turmeric, and green tea. These foods help your liver produce the enzymes and amino acids that aid in ridding itself of the toxins encountered daily.

Candida cleanse

Most people on Western diets have some level of Candida and yeast overgrowth. These fungi cause bloating, constipation, poor digestion, gas, hormonal imbalances, tiredness, and other ailments. A Candida cleanse is excellent for getting rid of live Candida organisms that live inside your gut and feed on your toxins as well as the yeast. You can simply take Candida cleansing tablets every night for a month or two, even during colonics. Of course, you will have to refrain from most sweets and sweet fruits during this period because Candida often feed on sugary foods. If you do not address Candida, your food cravings will continue.

Infrared sauna: skin cleansing

The cleansing treatments I just reviewed are the ones I recommend initially; a series of colonics comes first because it will take you into a new dimension of health. In addition, another fantastic way to cleanse other body organs is with sessions in a sauna. Your skin naturally accumulates toxins and waste, even while showering in highly chlorinated city water. Sweating in a sauna produces amazing health benefits. It helps stimulate the release of accumulated toxins. This in turn increases your metabolism, reduces your appetite, promotes weight loss, and increases metabolic rate, which is the energy you expend while resting.

The skin is the largest organ of your body. When you start cleansing more frequently, impurities will come out of your skin. One of the best ways to speed up the process is to allow your skin to sweat out the toxins. Saunas are the best way to do this—especially the infrared kind. Any sauna will help, but infrared saunas go much deeper and offer a cellular level of cleansing. Not only are they better than conventional saunas, but also they take less time. The deep heat penetration of infrared saunas removes not only toxins but also alcohol, nicotine, and metals. They also help cure chronic fatigue, promote muscle growth, and reduce cellulite. Also, you burn more calories (700 calories) sitting in this type of sauna for thirty minutes than you would running for a half hour.[3] If you don't always have time to exercise, you can relax in a sauna and read a book or listen to music. This will reap the same benefits as running or cardio while helping you de-stress.

There's more. Infrared saunas also help with blood circulation, leaving you more beautiful, youthful, and with glowing skin—a great help in reducing acne and even old scars. Many people have found pain relief for arthritis, back pain, muscle spasms, and headaches. Athletes use them to quickly recover from sprains, arthritis, muscle spasms, and back pain as the deep heat penetrates much deeper than a normal sauna.

Another benefit of infrared saunas is they increase oxygenation and remove radioactive residues. They also are good for chronic infections and have been found to be helpful to cancer patients. They help patients suffering from varicose veins, metal implants, hypertension, and diabetes where conventional saunas do not achieve these same results. And they require less energy and heat much faster than traditional saunas.

To increase the benefits of infrared sauna use, you can use a dry brush and brush off the skin before showering. This helps remove the toxins after your session and stimulates circulation. Skin brushing daily during your cleanse is also beneficial. Vigorously brush your skin before or during your shower or bath. Because the skin is the largest organ in your body, brushing has significant benefits, such as the direct improvement it produces in the lymphatic system, which directly strengthens your immune system by increasing the flow of the lymphocytes, or white blood cells, where it can fight toxins that are a threat to your health. Another benefit is unclogging skin pores, allowing your skin to "breathe" by ridding it of dead skin cells. This helps with decreasing odors and improving blood flow to the skin to increase perspiration and allowing toxins to exit more easily.

Because of their amazing health benefits now becoming known to more people, infrared saunas are more affordable than ever. You can usually purchase a portable, lightweight infrared sauna for less than $2,000. Whether you live in an apartment, mobile home, or a traditional house, infrared saunas are designed for storage in any housing situation—even outdoors. After experiencing their amazing benefits, I use one regularly now. This is one investment in your health that you can't afford to overlook. However, if you don't have access to the infrared kind, remember that any sauna will still aid good health.

Cleanses and Physical Activity

Depending on the type of cleanse you are doing, it can be unclear what type of physical activity you should be participating in to promote increased detoxification results. There are a few activities I recommend that you take on regularly throughout your cleanse: massages, walking outdoors, drinking lots of water, and rebounding. I will explain each in more detail to help you understand their detoxification-enhancing benefits.

Massage

While doing a series of colon and other cleanses, getting massages will greatly aid in pushing the toxins and lactic acid out of your system rapidly, plus they will increase circulation. Massage reduces stiffness. The best type of massages for stiffness that I recommend are deep tissue and Thai massage, but there are other types that are also beneficial. Some benefits to deep-tissue massage include the release of adhesions deep within the tissues that can block circulation and cause pain, limited movement, and inflammation. Deep-tissue massage can also help chronic pain and release toxic waste and lactic acid that would normally build up, especially when doing regular exercise. When your back is very sore for weeks and you just can't seem to shake it Thai massage which involves lots of stretching that you could not do on your own often loosens the tight muscles that could not otherwise be loosened. However, please check with your health care provider if this is a good choice for you.

Walking outdoors

During your cleansing routines you should strive to exercise a minimum of at least three times a week with some type of cardiovascular workout. Daily exercise will help you to cleanse much faster through sweating and improving blood circulation by elevating your heart rate. Exercise affects your hormones and body chemistry, which increases your overall sense of well-being. This provides more mental and emotional clarity and higher self-esteem. It is also a great stress reliever and relaxer. One of the best things you can do daily is to walk for an hour a day, or as much as you can initially, with that one-hour goal in mind. This helps cleanse every cell in your body and keeps your heart, blood, and many other organs clean. I recommend walking outdoors since getting fresh air has a significant impact on your body. You will feel more "grounded" when walking outdoors, since the earth is always moving and rotating. The opposite is true when you spend excessive amounts of travel time in a car or airplane. Once you arrive at your destination you feel unbalanced and unconnected. Walking outdoors keeps you in touch with the earth; the human body was made to walk.

Water

While cleansing, you need to drink a lot of water throughout each day. This will help push the toxins through your system rapidly as you detox simultaneously on many levels. Staying hydrated will give you more energy too. Your body is made primarily of water. A caution: you should use the best water possible, which means spring water or filtered water. If you can get a water filter for your home, that is even better; you will eliminate harmful chlorine and chemicals that enter your bloodstream every time you take a shower. And you will enjoy an unlimited supply of healthy drinking water.

Rebounding

The phenomenon known as "rebound exercise" is another method of internal cleansing that offers numerous health benefits for the human body. Labeled "the ultimate exercise for the new millennium" (also the title of a 2005 book by rebounding pioneer and former Olympic wrestler Albert Carter), rebounding involves working out on a mini-trampoline. One of its leading benefits is that it cleanses your lymphatic system by flushing away toxic substances. The body is always rounding these up from its normal processes, such as processing food wastes and filtering environmental pollutants—before they can form new waste by-products.

Dr. Morton Walker, the author of *Jumping for Health*, explains that "during rebounding arterial blood enters the capillaries in order to furnish the cells with fresh tissue fluid containing food and oxygen. The bouncing motion moves and recycles the lymph and the entire blood supply through the circulatory system many times during the course of the rebounding session. The feature of rebounding that sets it apart from all other exercises is that half of the time you do it you are not opposing gravity."[4] When you are bounced upward by the springs and mat of the quality rebounder, your body is not subject to the pull of gravity. Because of this action, each cell in the body and brain receives a positive stress. The joy of it is that you don't have to exert yourself to get these benefits. The eldest of the elderly, the handicapped, and the arthritic can do this, by doing a gentle, two-to-three minute "health bounce."

What is the "health bounce"? As Dr. Walker explains in his book, the lymphatic system is the "metabolic garbage can of the body. It rids you of toxins, such as dead and cancerous cells, nitrogenous wastes, fat, infectious viruses, heavy metals, and other material cast off by the cells."[5] The lymphatic fluid is a clear liquid that contains the body's T- and B-cells, which are cells that help the immune system ward off disease. When you rebound, you help your cells metabolize, cleanse, and renew. And you help your lymph system to pump and drain the body's waste. The cardiovascular hydraulics benefit too.

Linda Brooks—author of *Rebounding to Better Health*—writes, "Lymph is moved like a hydraulic pressure system. The lymph tubes are filled with one-way valves that only open up, or allow drainage toward the center of the body. When pressure below the valve is greater than above (as when you are moving downward on the rebounder), the valves are forced open so the fluid can flow."[6]

There are three primary ways for the lymph system to "pump" and cleanse:

1. Exercise, which helps muscular contraction

2. Massage (via movement) of the musculature or tissues, which serves to get it to pump back into the pulmonary circulation

3. Gravitational pressure with its resultant internal massage

Remarkably, rebounding provides all three ways of removing waste from cells. Medical researchers agree that aside from poor nutrition, the primary cause of fatigue, disease, cell degeneration, and premature aging is poor circulation to and from the tissues of the body. Rebounding gives you the most efficient forms of tissue oxygenation and blood circulation. Rebounding will help you to stimulate lymphatic circulation. This means the broken-down products of fat metabolism and toxins can drain out of your body through your liver and spleen. It can also help you rebuild cells that are stronger, healthier, more oxygen-enriched, and more resilient disease fighters.

Cleansing, or detoxing, is one of the best ways to reset your body and get it ready for a new healthy lifestyle. Cleanses accelerate healing, stamp out carb cravings, and refocus your mind to make it easier to adjust to new things. Once you have completed a cleanse, the next step is not to go back to how you lived, thought, and ate before the cleanse but to continue on in great health with the new habits you've become accustomed to.

In these next few chapters I am going to uncover some of nature's best kept secrets for weight loss, healing, beauty, and staying forever young and vibrant—super naturally.

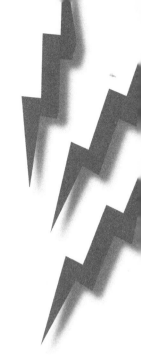

PART 2

THE POWER OF SUPER NATURAL FOOD

• Chapter 4 •

EAT YOUR WAY
TO A **HEALTHY WEIGHT**

Nothing tastes as good as being thin feels.[1]
—Elizabeth Berg,
author of *The Day I Ate Whatever I Wanted*

WITH NEARLY SEVEN out of every ten Americans over-weight and the worldwide obesity pandemic, weight loss has turned into an international obsession. According to Dr. Robert Lustig, whose "Sugar: The Bitter Truth" video is a YouTube sensation, the American diet industry alone generates $117 billion in annual revenues.[2] Everyone rushes to get in on the action, fueling a never-ending supply of advertisements for miracle weight-loss cures, slim-down plans, round-the-clock fitness centers, home exercise equipment, and on and on and on. The problem is, whether food- or fitness-based, most of these "cures" do not work. They are short-term solutions aimed at a long-term problem. The weight comes right back if you do not address the deeper issues behind weight gain. Once you tackle those causes, then you will not only lose weight, but also you will easily keep it off.

This is why I emphasize a lifestyle, not a diet. The more *Jump Start!* recommendations you incorporate into your daily life, the quicker the results. Try to incorporate these strategies into your lifestyle by adding at least one or two practices weekly until they develop into habits. As a health enthusiast, nutrition coach, researcher, motivational speaker, and life coach—and after years of research and experimentation using these principles and strategies—I have seen amazing results. In addition to my own life, I have observed them in many others' lives. Get ready to go from natural to super natural health while experiencing weight loss and recovering your life, joy, and energy!

Hindrances to Weight Loss

Before I share my weight-loss secrets, I need to address what causes the weight gain—and what *not to do*. The solution starts with the awareness that nonorganic food is the staple of most grocery stores, fast-food outlets, and chain restaurants. Their foods are loaded with chemicals, toxins, and processed junk that clog you up and cause food addictions (yes, you can be addicted, particularly to salt, sugar, and fat). False advertising, which seduces millions to consume nonnourishing, addictive foods, is a great contributor to the world's epidemic. To address this, your metabolism needs revving back up—naturally. Avoid some of these primary causes of weight gain, and you can start reversing the situation.

Clogged colon

Your colon gets clogged by dehydration (lack of water), lack of fiber, lack of walking and exercise, lack of enzymes in your food, and prescriptions and over-the-counter (OTC) drugs. Cleansing your colon is an absolute must! Remember: *if you do not experience at least three bowel movements daily, then you have a clogged colon.* If you ignore the problem, your metabolism will continue to decline and hunger pangs increase as your body signals it is not getting enough nutrients. Besides overeating, you will experience slower digestion and stomach bloat. As I mentioned previously, I recommend starting with a colon cleanse, followed by liver and Candida cleanses.

Clogged liver

Almost every overweight person who gets tested has a sluggish, clogged liver. The causes are many, but some primary culprits are a clogged colon, trans fats, prescription and OTC drugs, Candida yeast overgrowth, artificial sweeteners, and nonorganic, toxic foods. When your liver is clogged, your body rapidly stores high levels of body fat. Metabolism always slows, with the clogged liver contributing significantly to weight gain.

Candida

Most Westerners or those who consume a Western diet have some form of Candida. This causes cravings for foods like bread, pasta, cheese, and sweets. Candida blocks your colon, slowing metabolism and digestion and causing bloating, gas, and a protruding stomach. Once you take your first antibiotic, you destroy good bacteria, allowing bad bacteria like Candida yeast to grow at abnormal rates. Eventually, if not corrected, Candida turns into a fungus that spreads throughout your system.

Parasites

If you are overweight, it is quite likely you have parasites. Among other things, they are caused by a clogged colon, liver, Candida, heavy metal toxicity, and lack of nutrients. Parasites can live undetected in your body, robbing it of the essential nutrients by feeding off of the food you eat and leaving you with the fats and sugars to process for nutrition. This contributes to constantly feeling hungry and overeating. Parasites can contribute to symptoms such as stomach and intestinal issues (gas, bloating, diarrhea, chronic constipation, etc.); food allergies; heartburn; fatigue; skin disorders (dry skin and hair, allergies, itchy nose and skin in many areas, rashes, sores, etc.); mood and anxiety problems; and sleep disturbances. A parasite cleanse from your health food store can be used to rid your body of these.

Enzyme deficiency

Nonorganic foods or those that have been pasteurized or cooked—anything heated more than 180 degrees for at least thirty minutes—have no enzymes.[3] Even with vegetables, most people cook them and thus never get the enzymes and nutrients they need. (Some veggies are better slightly cooked or steamed, but they are exceptions.) Without enough enzymes you will experience trouble digesting food, low metabolism, frequent gas, constipation, and bloating. A lifestyle change to more raw foods, fresh, raw salads, and juicing raw veggies will help correct an enzyme deficiency. It will also promote easier digestion and better metabolism. As you start your diet, add some enzyme tablets to your meals. If you are overweight, past consumption of highly refined or pasteurized foods, prescription and OTC drugs, and a clogged liver and colon will hinder your ability to create enough enzymes to digest food properly. These supplements will help restore normalcy.

Stress

Ongoing stress will promote fat storage. No matter what your job description or lifestyle, there are things you can do to relieve stress, which I will review later in this book. For now, I will say that overexposure to cell phones, TV, electronic devices, and other currents going through your system will also stress your entire system.

Water deficiency

Most people are dehydrated from their failure to consume enough water. Frequent consumption of soft drinks and most popular caffeine drinks leads to more dehydration. Without pure drinking water your cells cannot properly hydrate, contributing to a slower metabolism. Those who drink tap water clog their system with phosphorus, chlorine, heavy metals, and toxins, to name a few. You need fresh water, or at least a filter at home.

Food additives

Eating a steady diet of nonorganic food means consuming pesticides, chemical fertilizers, herbicides, and thousands of artificial chemicals and antibiotics—especially if you live in North America. By copying this Western diet, many nations are quickly catching up to US obesity levels.

Fast food

If you hope to achieve super natural health and weight loss, you should avoid all fast-food restaurants, whether regional or national chains (especially in Westernized nations). Their foods are typically loaded with trans fats, highly processed sugars and high-fructose corn syrup, the flavor additive monosodium glutamate (MSG), artificial corn sweeteners, and nitrates. Meats and dairy from fast-food and many national chain restaurants are full of growth hormones, antibiotics, and other drugs. These highly processed foods are often microwaved, lack fiber, and are designed to ensure big profits. Companies create foods to increase hunger and cause addictions, which can lead to depression and weight gain.

Sodas and carbonated drinks

Carbonated drinks and sodas block calcium absorption, lowering metabolism and causing nutritional deficiencies. Sodas loaded with sugar are the worst offenders—and diet drinks are worse. A recent study published in the *American Journal of Clinical Nutrition* discovered diet sodas raised the risk of diabetes more than the fructose-sweetened kind and are more addictive because they are hundreds of thousands of times sweeter than regular sugar.[4]

Sugar and other sweeteners

An overload of sugar, desserts, high-fructose corn syrup, and other sweeteners promotes rapid weight gain. Whether regular or diet, sodas contain so much fructose or other sweeteners that your system goes into shock and overloads your system, causing high fat storage and insulin imbalance. Even artificial sweeteners—such as aspartame (NutraSweet) and sucralose (Splenda)—will slow your metabolism.

Lack of sleep

Over the past five decades Americans' average nightly sleep declined from more than eight hours to less than seven; at the same time the obesity rate climbed 30 percent. Less sleep means lower levels of leptin, the hormone that tells us we have eaten enough. "You're fighting against the tide to lose weight when you're sleep-deprived," says Dr. Amy Aronsky, medical director of The Center for Sleep Disorders in Portland, Oregon. "Good sleep is as important as a good diet and exercise when it comes to weight loss."[5]

By the way, according to Chinese medicine, the optimal bedtime is ten o'clock or earlier, since in deep sleep your liver starts to detox and cleanses itself between 10:00 p.m. and 2:00 a.m.[6] Lack of sleep or inconsistent sleep patterns hinder the cleansing process, which slows metabolism.

Lack of exercise

Poor circulation causes slower metabolism. Clogged arteries can cause circulation problems, with clogging originating with such factors as poor nutrition (an excess of trans fats), pasteurized dairy products, chlorine in your water, Candida, and heavy metals. Lack of exercise also contributes to poor circulation. The human body was made to walk, which is the most basic but effective method of improving circulation. In most countries people walk a minimum of five miles a day. However, in America the average person walks less than a tenth of a mile daily! Walking helps everything in your system circulate, which cleanses cells and rejuvenates your system.

Sunlight deficiency

Sunshine activates your metabolism and speeds it up. These natural rays also diminish depression and reduce stress.

Lack of sweating/perspiration

As I noted in the previous chapter, the skin is the body's largest organ and is designed to eliminate toxins on a regular basis. A lack of sweating clogs your lymphatic system and slows metabolism. As much as people love air-conditioning, we need to sweat to lose weight and toxins and achieve good health. Our cooling systems are another modern-world-lifestyle deficiency. Air-conditioning and a lack of regular sunlight lower metabolism.

Weak muscle mass

If you don't maintain normal muscle mass through exercise or physical labor, your metabolism will be slower. When you increase muscle mass, metabolism speeds up. If you increase muscle through exercise, this helps burn fat and increase metabolism—even while you sleep.

Whew! By now this long list may have worn you out, but it was necessary to educate you on some of the factors that contribute to weight gain. When your metabolism slows, it keeps you tired, groggy, and lethargic. When you feel this way, you lack passion and creativity. Once you make certain simple adjustments, you will be amazed at the weight you lose as you continue your journey from a natural to a super natural life.

Lose Weight Now

Adapting the following practices to your daily routine will increase your metabolism, burn fat, and help you shed weight. The more you do daily, the more weight you will lose as your health improves. I have listed them in order of importance.

Drink water

As soon as you awake in the morning, drink a large glass of water, preferably spring water or water filtered by reverse osmosis. Whether they know it or not, people who are overweight are always dehydrated. Drink 1.5 gallons of water throughout the day to flush out your system, taking care to avoid tap water. Its fluoride, chlorine, and other harmful chemicals can clog your system. If you drink bottled water, try to buy glass bottles as opposed to plastic bottles. Plastic often leaches into the water over time and is known to add unhealthy estrogen into your system.

Do cardio exercises

I suggest walking, running, or even a brisk swim for fifteen to twenty minutes before breakfast, and if possible, again before lunch. When you wake up, your body is in a semi-fasted state and will burn fat right away. Then, later in the day, walk for at least one hour outdoors. Or at least work toward to that goal by starting with twenty to thirty minutes, since anything you do daily will help. For those in better condition, running will increase weight loss.

Do rebounding

As I mentioned in chapter 3, rebounding is a great exercise because it stimulates the lymphatic system and releases helpful endorphins and other hormones. It is the only exercise that stimulates and exercises every cell simultaneously. It releases toxins, improves circulation, increases muscle tone and flexibility, and oxygenates the blood. Set up a rebounder in front of your TV or at your office and bounce for five to ten minutes once or twice daily. You will notice super natural physical, emotional, and mental health benefits—a great aid in weight loss.

Do a colonic cleanse

Why not make an appointment with a licensed colon therapist to get your health and weight-loss goals activated? Do anywhere from six to fifteen colonics during a thirty-day period. During the initial sessions the therapist will evaluate the number needed, which depends on how clogged you are and how fast you cleanse. To speed this up you can take a colon cleanse product in tablet form—before, during, or after. I recommend OxyPowder, which we carry at www.jumpstartthebook.com, or Raw Cleanse by Garden of Life.

Eat fat-busting fruits and veggies

Eat at least two organic apples daily. They are a super food, full of fiber, and will help fill you up. This reduces your appetite and helps cleanse the liver, gallbladder, and colon. In addition (unless a medication prohibits it), try to eat two grapefruits a day; they contain a lot of enzymes and burn and release fat stores. They also cleanse all the vital organs. Eat at least one organic avocado a day, either with a salad or alone. They have healthy fats that help you lose weight and give you a sense of fullness. Drink 2 teaspoons a day of extra-virgin raw coconut oil too. Among other things, it helps release fat cells, improves digestion, and speeds metabolism. Adding a tablespoon of raw organic apple cider vinegar will do the same.

Eat fiber

Increasing dietary fiber will drastically accelerate weight loss. Fiber has a long list of benefits, such as improving digestion, cleaning out toxins, helping turn back years of eating refined and processed foods, relieving constipation, and reducing appetite, to name a few. Take extra fiber during the first phase of your journey.

Drink tea

The best teas for providing natural energy and speeding up metabolism is green tea and Yerba Mate. Yerba Mate is my favorite; it increases energy but without the jitters or "crash" effects of coffee. It also stimulates the release of fat cells and reduces appetite. Drink at least one cup a day of both Yerba Mate and green tea. I like to mix mine together.

Eat 100 percent organic

Eating all organic is the best way to ensure nothing hinders you from reaching your weight-loss goals. You want fruits and vegetables free of chemicals. If you eat meat, make sure it is certified organic; if it isn't, it will likely contain growth hormones, antibiotics, and other animal drugs. This will clog your system and put animal hormones and chemicals into your body. This causes abnormal fat storage, weight gain, hormonal and menstrual problems in women, depression, and other problems. If you eat organic meat, include a large salad to speed up digestion.

Eat wild fish

Make sure your fish is wild, not farm-raised. Farm-raised fish live in small spaces and receive growth-inducing chemicals and drugs. They are often injected with chemical food dyes to make them look fresher. Farm-raised fish leads to weight gain and other hormonal imbalances.

Take supplements

Taken daily, these oils and supplements will speed up weight loss:

▶ Vitamin E: This vitamin improves liver and gall-bladder function; powerfully aids weight loss; creates young, fresh-looking skin; keeps arteries open; and promotes circulation. Look for natural vitamin E without synthetics.

▶ Omega-3: This essential fatty acid helps with fat burning, decreases appetite, improves liver and pancreas function, increases circulation and oxygenation in the body, and helps balance hormone levels.

▶ Acetyl L-carnitine: Used for fatty acid oxidation, this amino acid helps burn unwanted body fat. Fatty acids are one of the body's key energy sources; oxidation is the process by which they are broken down to create energy. This supplement will help burn off fat as fuel and energy.

▶ Alpha lipoic acid (ALA): ALA mimics insulin, which may enhance the body's sensitivity to insulin. This helps improve your ability to build lean body mass and reduce fat, which is good if trying to add healthy muscle mass. It also works with creatine to promote energy and improve general metabolism. The body produces ALA in very small quantities. So if you want the best possible therapeutic benefits, consider a supplement. ALA works best in conjunction with vitamins C and E and contains powerful antiaging and antioxidant qualities. Anyone with diabetes should only use this supplement with a doctor's approval.

Use a shower filter

Most municipal water is loaded with fluoride, chlorine, heavy metals, and other chemicals. Showering in it means absorbing more toxins than drinking eight glasses. Hot showers in such water create steam-releasing, poisonous gases, which you inhale and get into your lungs and skin. The best step is to buy a high-quality filter so you shower in pure, clean water. It will boost your energy levels and get rid of any dry skin problems, which will give you an improved sense of well-being.

Get a massage

If you can afford them, I recommend regular massages during your first phase of cleanses and diet changes—as often as possible. They will speed up weight loss and help flush out toxins and lactic acid. A deep-tissue massage is best, since it goes deeper on a cellular level. However, any massage is beneficial and can influence your ability to control or lose weight. A massage improves circulation, the supply of nutrition to the muscles, and tissue metabolism. It maximizes the supply of nutrients and oxygen through increased blood flow, which helps muscles to grow and burn more calories. During and after exercise, such waste products as lactic and carbonic acid build up in muscles. Increased circulation to these muscles helps to eliminate toxic buildup caused by these waste products and shortens muscles' recovery time.

Get some sun

Lack of exposure to sunlight slows your metabolism, leading to weight gain, possible depression, and increased appetite and overeating. Doctors recommend ten to twenty minutes a day of sun on your face and body. Moderate sun exposure—with proper protection, depending on your skin type—will boost your immune system and ward off sickness and certain types of cancers.

Infrared sauna

The ancients of Finland are credited for the invention of the sauna for healing and cures in ancient times. Sweating in a sauna will release fat cells and increase metabolism while releasing toxins, reducing appetite, helping with arthritis and muscle pain, decreasing depression, and relaxing your mind and body. As I mentioned in the previous chapter, you can lose more calories sitting in the infrared sauna than running for the same length of time, but you need to do both for different reasons. Sauna use helps to break up fat-containing cellulite, which are more stubborn fat cells. They can melt away in an infrared sauna. These saunas also deeply cleanse skin, often healing acne, boosting the immune system, and providing a host of other benefits.

Applying as many of these items to your lifestyle as possible will increase your weight-loss results. The first thing to do is to get cleansed. Then eat organic, drink fresh water, and get some exercise. Now you are on your way to super natural health!

But as with any diet plan—including the one listed in this book—check with your physician before beginning it.

• Chapter 5 •

ULTIMATE HEALING FOODS

Let food be thy medicine and medicine by thy food.[1]
—Ancient Greek physician Hippocrates

R AW FOODS REPRESENT amazing medicine for the body and provide mind-boggling levels of energy, health, and vitality. I know this from past experience, thanks to these foods bringing healing from a severe attack on my immune system. While not sleeping enough, for a few weeks I also over-exerted myself at work and during exercise. Suddenly I grew very weak and developed a severe sore throat, with bumps on my head and near my ears—the result of swollen lymph nodes. I sweated a lot too. Basically, my immune system needed a major reboot, and I needed a lot of rest. For maximum healing I only drank miracle foods. Why? When you refrain from eating, your body focuses all its energies on healing instead of digestion. That is why you want to liquefy these foods in a blender or juicer. Here are some miracle foods that helped me to quickly cleanse my body and heal by acting as natural antibiotics.

Rapid Immune System Fixes

► One ripe orange habanera pepper (or a ripe jala-peño): You will feel this cleanse you as fire-like sensations course through your body, killing bacteria and viruses. It also will start to clear out nasal passages of mucus almost immediately.

► Two cloves of garlic and one slice of ginger: Garlic and ginger are natural antibiotics that boost a weakened immune system. Ginger also helps reduce swelling in the throat. These are "power twins" for fighting infections.

► Six figs: Figs are amazing at dissolving mucus and cleansing the gastrointestinal tract, helping to detox your body.

► One handful of parsley or kale: Both of these are rich in iron, which builds strong red-blood corpuscles.

► Two organic apples (or four organic pears): Apples and pears contain pectin, which helps to remove toxins. They help with bowel movements, which drains the lymphatic system and alleviates swelling in a sore throat and tonsils.

► One ounce organic, cold-pressed, extra-virgin olive oil: Olive oil helps to build strong white blood corpuscles.

As a public speaker, I address audiences across America and around the world. On the rare occasion when a sore throat strikes, it is imperative that I get healed—ASAP! Going the healthy route, I create a powerful, miracle tea that alleviates the pain by stopping by a health food store for the ingredients and picking up warm water at a deli.

Colloidal silver

Another way to boost your immune system is to take powerful natural supplements. One of my favorites is colloidal silver, a dietary supplement made of pure silver and distilled water. Throughout the centuries it fulfilled multiple functions.

Hundreds of years ago, during the origins of the pharmaceutical market, people used natural products to prevent infections instead of turning to antibiotics, which have polluted our bodies and water (not to mention creating more "superbugs" that can prove nearly impossible to fight). Dating back much farther in history, colloidal silver was a leading health product, due to its efficiency in supporting the immune system. With the expansion of the medical world—and, consequently, the pharmaceutical industry—its use did not increase. Yet, ironically, laboratories and specialists discovered new uses for this product, such as stress relief, a skin conditioner, and enhanced physical performance.

The rich concentration of silver molecules in colloidal silver essentially destroys bacteria and viruses and keeps the immune system safe and sound. Moreover, products based on colloidal silver are nontoxic. Nor do they lose power to act when in contact with other antibiotics or medical treatments. The silver component has been proven to be compatible with the human body and no tolerance limit found to prevent its use.

Furthermore, unlike antibiotic medications, colloidal silver does not require long-term treatment. This happens because silver particles destroy viruses and germs from initial contact. Because of this, bacteria and other microorganisms do not have time to develop a firewall against these particles. With outbreaks of strange viruses occurring regularly, this is one of the best ways to stay healthy and protected.

Echinacea and goldenseal

This is another "dynamic duo" of the herb kingdom that I take when traveling or at home if I feel something coming on. The extract is helpful for naturally boosting and fortifying the defense ("immune") system. It purifies the blood and lymph fluids, strengthens and tones all the major organs and glands, and helps repair damage to the major eliminative channels by cleansing the tissues.

Astragalus

The complex polysaccharides found in astragalus herbs appear to act as an immunomodulator, a fancy medical term for treating disease by inducing, enhancing, or suppressing an immune response. Immunomodulators possess the natural ability to increase the body's production of messenger cells that regulate the immune system. The overall effect is a more efficient immune system. Studies on astragalus indicate that it can prevent white blood cell numbers from falling in patients receiving chemotherapy and radiotherapy. It can also elevate antibody levels in healthy people.

Reishi mushroom

Though used in traditional Chinese medicine for at least two thousand years, only recently has the reishi mushroom received much attention for to its apparent immune-enhancing activities. Studies have shown that reishi may transform many components of the immune system, including NK (natural killer) cells. Moreover, one study concluded that reishi's effect on such immune-related cells as T and B cells yielded further evidence that reishi's value comes from its ability to enhance immunity response.[2]

Other Remedies and Recipes

Healing a sore throat

6 to 8 oz. warm water (preferably fresh spring water)

Juice of ½ lemon

A few cut-up pieces of fresh raw ginger or 1 Tbsp. ginger powder

1 tsp. or Tbsp. of raw honey

Mix ingredients together and drink.

Natural flu and cold medicine

Influenza and colds are common. While their appearance sends many people running to the pharmacy, I have noticed that as you cleanse your body, it does not respond well to pharmaceutical medicines that end up clogging your system. Raw natural foods act as a potent source of healing without any side effects. Below is what I do at the first signs of oncoming flu or cold. Try drinking the following blend on an empty stomach three times a day, replacing meals for a few days. Or try it while fasting for at least twenty-fours and see how quickly you heal.

4 oranges, peeled, but keeping white pith (oranges and papayas are excellent antioxidants)

1 papaya, skinned, with seeds removed (Both oranges and papayas will cleanse toxicity, which is what leads to a weakened immune system. They also help cleanse your intestinal tract and are full of calcium and rich in vitamin A, beta-carotene, and vitamin C.)

6 figs, soft, with stem removed (these are one of the best mucus dissolvers)

Optional: 1 hot pepper, jalapeño, or orange habanera pepper, to cleanse the sinus cavities and fight bacteria (Hot peppers contain phyto-antibiotics, which wipe out bacteria-causing sickness.)

Optional: 1 avocado, for added thickness to offset the hot peppers

Super-food energy blend ("Maca Chaca" Drink)

For those who would love a meal replacement that is full of energy, strength, and stamina and that tastes good, here is what I drink almost daily! It starts with wild young coconut water. You can either buy a fresh coconut and use the water and flesh, or you can buy coconut water at the health food store with the flesh to save time (though wild is always better.) Coconut water hydrates your body more than plain water and cools the body, especially in hot or tropical locations. Then add the following:

- ► *1 small handful of goji berries:* These are the highest antioxidant energy food on the planet because they grow in the highest altitudes on the earth—places like Tibet—and are able to withstand harsh climates where almost nothing else grows. They contain at least eighteen amino acids and are a complex protein, as well as an excellent source of minerals. Plus, they taste great!

- ► *1 tablespoon of raw chocolate powder:* This type of chocolate is full of raw nutrients and helps with weight loss since it inhibits appetite and tastes awesome! You can replace raw chocolate powder with raw chocolate nibs.

- ► *1 teaspoon or tablespoon of maca:* This food helps to regulate hormones, increase energy, and increase testosterone in men and progesterone in women. Maca is rich in minerals and increases vigor and affects your mood positively.

- ► *1 teaspoon or tablespoon of spirulina:* This has one of the highest concentrations of natural protein (along with chlorella) on the planet! The ancient peoples of Mexico and Africa consumed this algae for thousands of years.

Benefits of Goji Berries

- 500 times more vitamin C by weight than oranges
- Has vitamin E, which is nearly unheard of in fruits
- More beta-carotene than carrots
- Contains B vitamins
- Helps increase testosterone and libido
- Contains nineteen amino acids, which include eight essential amino acids
- Contains twenty-one trace minerals, which include zinc, calcium, and selenium
- Contains beta-sitosterol, which aids in lowering cholesterol and improves sexual health
- Has antibacterial and antifungal properties
- Has essential fatty acids such as omega-6
- Has anticancer properties

The Power of Spirulina

The original super food, spirulina is a single-celled, blue-green algae that contains ten vitamins, eight minerals, and eighteen amino acids, both essential and nonessential. It contains vegetable protein of 65 to 71 percent, which is twelve to fifteen times more than that found in steak. In addition, it is five times easier to digest than the protein in meat or soy products. It helps reduce weight and helps combat many allergies, vision problems, carbohydrate disorders, anemia, and other diseases. It also has many beneficial enzymes. This "super" algae gets its deep blue-green color from the chlorophyll and phycocyanin. The green pigment stems from chlorophyll, which is sometimes called "green blood" because it is so similar to hemoglobin.

Spirulina facts

In 1989 the National Cancer Institute announced sulfolipids from blue-green algae such as spirulina were remarkably active in test tube experiments against the AIDS virus. Other research from 1993 to 1995 showed the natural polysaccharides in spirulina strengthened the immune system by increasing T-cell counts; these are cells that help direct the immune system's response to infection or malignancy. These polysaccharides also raised disease resistance in chickens, fish, and mice. Spirulina contains helpful glycolipids too. In recent years the animal feed industry has embraced spirulina as a probiotic to replace overused antibiotics in animal feed.

In 1994 the Russian government awarded a patent for the use of spirulina as a medical food for reducing allergic reactions from radiation in children exposed to hazardous material after the Chernobyl nuclear plant disaster in the Ukraine in 1986. During the aftermath of the disaster, a dose of 5 grams of spirulina for forty-five days successfully fought radiation poisoning.[3] By now you may not be surprised to learn that spirulina is the world's highest beta-carotene food—ten times more concentrated than carrots. So even if you don't eat the recommended four to nine daily servings of fruits and vegetables (most people eat only one or two), you can obtain natural beta-carotene insurance from spirulina to help support your body's defenses.

In addition, spirulina has gamma-linolenic acid (GLA), a rare essential fatty acid that is a key to good health. In mother's milk GLA helps develop healthy babies. However, standard Western diets of processed foods contain no GLA. Since studies show nutritional deficiencies can block GLA production in your body, a good dietary source is vital.[4] Spirulina is one of the few whole foods with GLA, which is helpful in fighting such sicknesses as heart disease, arthritis, skin disorders, and allergies. I always mix spirulina into my raw food smoothies. It is great for those who want to cut down on meats, or for vegetarians and raw foodists, since it is the most potent plant protein.

Spirulina contains cobalamin (a type of B_{12}), which is one of the most difficult of all vitamins to obtain from a plant source. Spirulina contains 250 percent more B_{12} than beef liver.[5] How's that for effectiveness?

Spirulina contains eight essential amino acids: isoleucine, leucine, lysine, methionine, phenylalanine, threonine, tryptophan, and valine. These acids perform such tasks as growth, increasing muscular energy, stimulating brain function, contributing to improved mental capacity, metabolizing fats and lipids to maintain a healthy liver, aiding digestion, and enhancing emotional stability.

The ten nonessential amino acids in spirulina are alanine, arginine, aspartic acid, cystine, glutamic acid, glycine, histidine, proline, serine, and tyrosine. Don't let the "nonessential" label fool you, though. Among the benefits these substances provide are helping strengthen cell walls, keeping the blood clean, transforming carbohydrates into energy, stabilizing blood sugar, and alleviating food allergies.

Spirulina's eight minerals include potassium, calcium, zinc, magnesium, selenium, iron, phosphorus, and pyridoxine (or B_6). Why are they important? To name a few: Potassium helps maintain the body's fluid level balance and control pressure, and—like calcium and magnesium—support nerve and muscle functions. Zinc boosts the immune system and has antioxidant properties. Magnesium aids healthy bone growth and functioning of the nerves and muscles; it may also prevent migraines and high blood pressure. Although many plants contain iron, the body doesn't readily absorb it. The iron in spirulina is highly absorbable, strengthening blood and muscle cells.

Chlorella Perfection

As impressive as spirulina is, chlorella has been touted as the perfect whole food. Aside from being a complete protein and containing all the B vitamins, vitamin C, vitamin E, and major minerals (with zinc and iron in amounts large enough to be considered supplementary), its benefits include improving the immune system and digestion; cleaning the body of toxins, mercury, and heavy metals; accelerating healing; protecting against radiation; aiding in the prevention of degenerative diseases; helping treat Candida; and relieving arthritis pain. Plus, because of its nutritional content, it aids in weight loss.

If that weren't enough, chlorella contains ten to one hundred times more chlorophyll than leafy green vegetables. It is grown in a controlled environment where minerals are added to optimize it for human consumption. Its small size requires centrifuge harvesting and special processing to improve the digestibility of its tough outer wall, which makes it more expensive than spirulina. However, chlorella's cell wall binds to heavy metals, pesticides, and carcinogens such as PCBs and escorts the toxins out of the body, making it a particularly valuable supplement.

I find chlorella especially helpful during a cleanse. It is especially useful during colonics as it attaches to the cell walls of your intestines, pulling out impacted fecal matter and hard-to-remove toxins. Chlorella is probably one of the best natural defenses against cancer. I take it daily in tablet form (especially when I travel). There are several papers on the prevention and/or inhibition of cancer using chlorella as well as documentation of its DNA repair mechanism.[6] However, be careful to use it as directed.

Organic Pure Grass Juices

Organic pure grass juices like wheatgrass, barley grass, and alfalfa deliver high concentrations of valuable nutrients. They include such things as vitamins, minerals, naturally occurring enzymes, and chlorophyll. Moreover, their alkalinizing effects will promote healthy pH balance in the body. Typical diets that include processed foods—white flour, sugar, coffee, and soft drinks—cause a pH imbalance in the body, resulting in the body becoming too acidic. Too much acid in one's body will decrease the body's ability to absorb nutrients and minerals, decrease the energy production in cells, and make the body more susceptible to illness and fatigue. Therefore, maintaining a healthy pH balance is necessary for optimal health.

While many of these grasses are helpful, it is worth pointing out the powerful benefits of wheatgrass:

Blood benefits

Wheatgrass and organic pure grass juice tablets may help clean the blood of impurities, as well as increase the red blood cell count and lower blood pressure. Wheatgrass may also encourage the body's metabolism and enzymes to work more efficiently and increase blood flow.

Stomach disorders

Wheatgrass tablets have been used to treat diarrhea, constipation, colitis, and certain ulcers. Wheatgrass is also suggested for stomach pain and distress.

Turning back the clock

Wheatgrass tablets may help restore gray hair to its natural color. It is also used as a kind of youth tonic to help keep the body young, alert, energized, and fit. Some say it enhances fertility in both men and women.

Anti-inflammatory

Wheatgrass tablets contain the enzyme SOD, which claims to reduce the harsh side effects of radiation. This enzyme is also useful in protecting cell damage, especially after a heart attack.

Fight tumors and toxins

Wheatgrass tablets may be able to ward off toxins and fight tumors. The compounds found in wheatgrass help cleanse the blood and counteract toxins that may invade the body. Because I travel often, I don't always have the time to make the juice, nor do I always like the taste of liquid grass juices like wheatgrass. However, since I love the incredible results it produces in my immune system, I take them in organic tablet form.

Healing Power of Coconuts

Coconuts are one of the most amazing super foods on the planet. I use coconut water daily as the water base to all my shakes and raw drinks since it is the most complete hydrating liquid a human can consume. With the exception of vitamins B_6 and B_{12}, the water and flesh from young coconuts contain the full range of B vitamins. These are essential for providing energy, as they break down carbohydrates and proteins. They also support nervous system function and, interestingly, the muscle tone of the stomach. Young coconut water is also high in minerals, particularly calcium (for bones), magnesium (for the heart), and potassium (for muscles).

Coconut water is more nutritious than whole milk—less fat and NO cholesterol!

It is better than processed baby milk and contains lauric acid, which is present in human mother's milk. It is also naturally sterile—water permeates through the filtering husk! Its most amazing benefit is its ability to serve as a universal donor, since it is very similar in make up to blood plasma. Some nations use it for blood transfusions when they run out of blood donors! In fact, it was regularly used during World War II for wounded soldiers if blood plasma ran low.[7]

Coconut water is a natural isotonic beverage—the same level we have in our blood. I have found that it is more hydrating than water or any electrolyte sports drink. Indeed, this is how many survive on coconuts in hot, jungle-like tropical climates. It not only hydrates you but also cools down the body temperature while energizing you. My favorite coconut drink, which can be purchased with or without the coconut flesh in the water, can be found in many healthy food stores, such as Whole Foods or New Frontiers. You can buy all natural and canned varieties to take with you on trips.

Coconuts also help with weight loss. The effect on your thyroid from coconuts is shocking; studies have shown that they can boost thyroid function significantly.[8] Having an efficient thyroid is essential for our bodies to carry out several functions, including boosting our metabolism and energy production. In the 1940s farmers tried coconut oil to fatten their animals but discovered that it made them lean and active and increased their appetite. Whoops! Then they tried an anti-thyroid drug. Though it fattened their livestock with less food, it had a drawback: the drug proved carcinogenic (cancer-causing). In the late 1940s, farmers learned that they could achieve the same anti-thyroid effect by feeding animals soybeans and corn.[9]

Coconut is also a potent antibacterial and antifungal agent. It is a great cleanser of our gut and is something that can help heal the gut, should problems such as leaky gut syndrome occur. Plus, coconuts will help your body fight off infection, so it is great to eat when you feel weak or as if some strange virus is attacking you. The body converts it to monolaurin, which fights off infections (viral or bacterial).

It keeps getting better—coconuts have been proven to have anti-cancer effects, especially of the colon and breast. This is due to the oil's protective nature and ability to safeguard the body from infection while cleansing your system.

Supplements That Heal

Saw palmetto

One supplement that men should definitely include in their arsenal is saw palmetto. This popular "men's herb" is used primarily as a treatment for an enlarged prostate. As many as 50 percent of men experience symptoms of an enlarged prostate by age sixty. One man in six will receive a prostate cancer diagnosis during his lifetime, but only one man in thirty will die of this disease.[10] Still, prostate cancer is the second leading cause of cancer death in men in the United States. Time and money invested now will pay huge dividends later.[11]

Coenzyme Q_{10}

Found in every cell of your body, coenzyme Q_{10} (CoQ_{10}) is a similar to a vitamin. It is not only found in every cell, but it is also *needed by every cell.* Among its key benefits are helping treat congestive heart failure and improving nerve function. It is fundamental to energy production at the cellular level by strengthening the mitochondria (the part of the cell responsible for creating energy). CoQ_{10} is an important element for creating cellular energy. It provides protection against strokes, improves blood pressure, and—due to its potent antioxidants—improves skin by slowing down the aging process. It also has the capability of destroying free radicals. One study suggests it may help improve glucose control in type 2 diabetics,[12] while another study said that a 400-milligram dosage helped to promote cancer remission, including prostate and breast cancer.[13]

Transforming Your Body

The human body is the most amazing creation. Our bodies are always re-creating themselves—each and every day. Many in health and science fields have stated that 98 percent of the atoms in our bodies are replaced every year.[14] When you change your eating and living habits by eating organic, raw, green, alkalizing, and highly mineralized foods, you can speed up this process. You can alter your bones, skin, hair, weight, and internal organs, re-creating and rebuilding your atomic structure into what the Creator intended humans to look and feel like.

In this process you will also be rebuilding and helping to release and activate the most important aspect of your being—namely, your spiritual as well as mental, emotional, and physical states, which are all interconnected. So go ahead and eat your way to a new you!

•Chapter 6•

NATURE'S BEST-KEPT
BEAUTY SECRETS

Don't be afraid to be amazing.[1]
—Storyteller Andy Offutt Irwin

AMAZING. THAT INNER desire to look great, achieve great things, and—most of all—feel amazing burns within everyone's heart. Yet you cannot achieve such success just by wishing it would happen. Caring for yourself so you radiate from your inner joy that reflects your outward appearance takes effort, yet it is quite possible.

Six Super Foods for Gorgeous Younger-Looking Skin

Here are the six "secret" foods emperors, kings, actors, and models have used to fuel their bodies for thousands of years. For you, right here and now, they are no longer a secret. These beautifying foods are at your fingertips in your grocer's produce section, health food store, or local farmers market. You can enjoy them directly or juice them.

1. Cucumbers

The Roman emperor Tiberius loved cucumbers so much that, according to Pliny, he was never without them.[2] Though native to western Asia, they were also popular with the Egyptians, Greeks, Romans, and Sumerians. Alexander the Great—a king of Macedon, a state in northern ancient Greece—introduced them to Europe. Then legendary Italian explorer Christopher Columbus carried them to the newly discovered Americas in the late 1400s.[3] Cucumbers are one of the most beautifying foods available, especially if you blend them with celery and apples as a juice drink. They are an excellent source of silica, which is a trace mineral that contributes to the strength of connective tissues. Connective tissue is what holds your body together.

Cucumbers are also effective when used for various skin problems, including swelling under the eyes and sunburn. They also contain ascorbic and caffeic acids, which prevent water retention. That may explain why, when applied topically, cucumbers are often helpful for swollen eyes, burns, and dermatitis. Cucumbers have a high water and low sugar content. This makes them perfect as a beautifying food—inside and out, especially for skin. Their natural saltiness helps transport their juice into the tissues, thus hydrating the body at a deeper level. They also are a great kidney cleanser. Their primary enzyme, erepsin, helps to digest foods and proteins, and aids in killing tapeworms. The silicon and chlorophyll in the cucumber's skin greatly improve skin complexion. (Note: If you eat the skin, make sure it is organic.) Cucumbers are a perfect food as they are hydrating, low calorie, alkaline, high energy, cleansing, and skin beautifying.

A Recipe for Clear Skin

Often, the secret to clear skin is perfecting your diet. Certain foods are better for your complexion than others, so make sure you incorporate plenty of skin-clearing ingredients into your daily diet. Try out this salad recipe that combines four essential foods for clear skin!

SUPER SKIN COMPLEXION SALAD

How to make it: combine lettuce, cucumbers, celery, and papayas. Optional: Add avocado for added taste and a sense of fullness.

Why it's great for your skin: Celery cleans the skin cells of dirt and removes skin oils, fights acne, and reduces scars. Cucumbers hydrate your skin due to their high water and silica content, which greatly enhances skin tone. Papayas not only taste great, but they also enhance skin beauty due to their high collagen and vitamin C content. Finally, avocados reduce wrinkles and create a more toned skin due to high collagen production from their healthy oils.

2. Papayas

The beautifying effects of miraculous papayas include enhancing skin beauty, nail strength, and hair luster. Papayas contain large quantities of calcium and vitamin A, as well as high levels of collagen-healing vitamin C. Besides eating them to help prevent acne, you can also fight acne by applying a mask using the fleshy side of a green papaya skin. Papayas are one of the best foods for digestion. They may also help reduce the risk of heart attacks, certain strokes, and arteriosclerosis—partially due to their carpaine, an alkaloid compound. Papayas contain antitumor and anticancer properties;[4] due to their low sugar content (recommended for fighting cancer), half-ripe papayas are often prescribed for rawfood eaters. Also, their higher enzyme content helps with weight loss and flatulence.[5] When I surf in Hawaii, my absolute favorite breakfast is Hawaiian papayas right before I go ride some waves.

3. Celery

Celery is especially great for your skin as it can clean the cells and remove dirt and oil from skin. It can help you both fight against acne and dilute acne scarring. It is extremely efficient for people who want to lose weight and maintain their health. The exceptional benefits of celery have been recognized for centuries by ancient medical practitioners. Hippocrates, the father of medicine, claimed that celery played a major role in calming the nerves.[6] The 1897 Sears catalog even offered a nerve tonic made from celery.[7] Celery neutralizes the organism, promotes the proper functioning of the immune system, purifies our bodies, and keeps them in balance.

Furthermore, it is a great source of calcium, which helps to build strong teeth and bones. What's more, celery provides your body vitamin A and is a great source of B vitamins, such as B_1, B_2, and B_6. The latter give you energy for a fresh start to the day. It is also high in such nutrients as magnesium, iron, folic acid, and potassium.[8] It contains plenty of water too, which provides proper hydration for blood cells. Due to its high water and potassium content, celery is used for cosmetic purposes and is highly effective for treating dry, dehydrated skin.[9] Celery rehydrates the body and helps to maintain a healthy libido.[10]

A Radiation-Fighting Recipe

Since the Japanese nuclear meltdown that followed the 2011 earthquake and tsunami, people have grown concerned about increased radiation exposure. What many often don't realize is that we are exposed to radiation on a daily basis via our cell phones, X-ray systems, airport body scanners, and many other factors. However, certain foods can shield us from radiation exposure. Try putting them all together in this tasty salad recipe.

Lettuce

Cilantro

Powdered spirulina

Avocado

Pear slices

Kelp

Miso

Mix all ingredients into a salad, adding vinegar and oil or your own healthy vinaigrette dressing.

Why is it great for radiation protection?

- Cilantro will move heavy metals and radioactive material out of the cells and into the detoxification pathways.
- Spirulina reduces the effects of radiation.
- Pears are high in pectin; pectin is one of the most effective means of protecting against radiation when consumption of contaminated food becomes unavoidable.

- Kelp contains organic iodine, which will saturate the thyroid, preventing radioactive iodine from being absorbed.
- "Miso is effective for detoxifying your body of radiation. During World War II, two hospitals that were located side by side got hit with atomic radiation. In one hospital people consumed miso, and all of them survived. Many people in the other hospital who did not take miso died."[11]
- While avocados are optional, they add taste and round out the meal with healthy oils and fats.

4. Avocados

Despite the bad rap they sometimes get for having too much fat, avocados are amazingly healthy. Yes, they do contain up to 15 percent of the daily recommended amount of fat. However, it is good fat—the polyunsaturated and monounsaturated fat that helps to moisturize your skin and keep you feeling satisfied. You can apply it to your face in mask form, which does wonders for your skin, so why not try eating it to see its other benefits? Eaten in moderation, the monounsaturated fats you ingest will give you clear, soft, and smooth skin.

Avocados contain folate, which helps blood formation and is essential for cell regeneration. The oil from avocados aids in triggering the production of collagens. So incorporating more avocados into your diet will mean less wrinkles and a more even, toned skin appearance. Avocados are rich in potassium (60 percent more than bananas[12]), vitamin A, vitamin E (an effective, fat-soluble antioxidant vital to the normalcy of our body's functions), and B vitamins, which help with metabolism and energy levels. The brighter the fruit, the more beta-carotene it contains, so look for vibrant green ones that are slightly soft to the touch. If your favorite market or health food store only stocks harder, unripe avocados, just ripen them in a brown bag for two to three days.

5. Watermelon

Watermelon's red color comes from the lycopene in it (which is also found in tomatoes). Lycopene has been associated with lowering the risk of some cancers and protects the skin from oxygen damage. Oxygen damage can weaken the epidermis and make it a thriving environment for acne-causing bacteria to thrive. Watermelon has many other beauty benefits as well. Its juice protects skin from the sun's harmful rays, can act as a natural exfoliant on skin (which helps to clear it of blemishes), and can aid in regenerating new skin cells.[13]

6. Onions

While onions may not be the most romantic choice when it comes to your breath, after you hear about their benefits, you may decide that a few missed kisses will be worth the sacrifice. Besides adding flavor to food, onions' therapeutic properties might interest you more than their taste. Onions have antibacterial and antifungal aspects that ultimately bring beauty to your skin. They are full of sulfur, containing more than one hundred sulfur-containing compounds (these compounds are why we shed tears when cutting onions). They help cleanse the skin by purifying the liver. A cleaner liver will ease food digestion and keep blood flowing properly. Since one cup of onions will provide 20 percent of the recommended daily intake of chromium,[14] a bacteria-reducing mineral, onions aid in the battle against acne as well.

Magnificent Minerals for
Healthy Hair, Nails, and Teeth

Silicon

Silicon is a mineral with remarkable healing, regenerative, and beautifying properties. It is highly concentrated in hair and nails and is also present in skin, teeth, connective tissue, muscles, bones, cartilage, and lungs. Silicon has the incredible ability to transform into calcium. Therefore, a silicon-rich diet leads to an increase in bone mineral density and beautiful teeth and jaw formation while helping reduce tooth and gum decay.

Studies have shown that the oral and external application of silicon improves the condition of aging skin, hair, and nails in women.[15] Silicon increases the thickness and strength of skin, smooths out wrinkles, and gives hair and nails a healthier appearance. Plus, it plays a vital role in the formation of connective tissue. Consequently it helps to maintain the elastic quality of the skin, tendons, and, generally, of cell walls.

You can increase your intake of silicon by consuming these silicon-rich foods: cucumbers, bell peppers, and tomatoes (eat all three with the skin, making sure they are organic), radishes, romaine lettuce, marjoram, and nopal cactus (or prickly pear cactus).

Zinc

Zinc is necessary for the proper functioning of several enzymatic functions important for healthy skin. It is essential for a beautiful skin complexion, since it is necessary for the functioning of enzymes that digest damaged collagen and build new collagen.

Zinc also promotes cell division, repair, and growth. It helps the lymphatic system to oxygenate the tissues and eliminate wastes properly. In addition, it works synergistically with other minerals and vitamins. For instance, in combination with sulfur and vitamin A, zinc helps to build strong hair.

You can naturally increase the levels of zinc in your body by eating—preferably raw—the following zinc-rich foods: pumpkin seeds, pecans, cashews, sunflower seeds, sesame seeds, coconuts, and pine nuts. Besides eating the raw organic foods that contain zinc, I like to take natural zinc supplements to make sure I have the right amount in my system.

Beautifying Supplements

DMAE

A liquid organic compound, DMAE's (short for dimethylamino-ethanol) most promising benefit is promoting healthy skin. It does this by stopping the body's process of manufacturing arachidonic acid, which is a substance that can lead to wrinkles and aging of the skin. And it reduces the appearance of wrinkles, age spots, and other problems that come with age. Another function of DMAE is the improvement of concentration and memory, as well as treating autism, memory deficits, depression, and dementia. It may treat sleep problems, Alzheimer's, and ADHD. DMAE can counter depression by lifting one's mood level to more positive levels and raise and improve cognitive functions (such as memory and concentration). DMAE can even increase intelligence.[16]

While the body produces small amounts, for many people supplementation may be necessary. It is best to check with your doctor if you think you need to take DMAE—although you can buy it without a prescription. Physicians closely watching patients on DMAE have reported that such people are more upbeat and have greater positive mental acuity.[17] Also, people taking it often report sleeping more deeply and having much more energy when awake.

Among food sources of DMAE are oily fish, such as sardines, anchovies, squid, and salmon.

MSM (methylsulfonylmethane)

Made of sulfur, MSM benefits skin, hair, and nails, and has a beautifying effect on them as it smooths the skin. Its collagen-building effects strengthen hair and nails and cause acceleration of hair growth, which promotes luster. Sulfur is an essential component of all connective tissue. It is also vital in the formation of keratin, collagen, and elastin, which give flexibility, tone, and strength to muscles, bones, joints, internal membranes, skin, hair, and nails. Sulfur can clear up acne, sometimes in a matter of weeks. Its effects are accelerated by adding vitamin C, such as camu camu powder or capsules.

MSM is also a free-radical scavenger. It can give a relief from swelling, inflammation, pain, and symptoms of arthritis; research has shown that sufferers' conditions improved by taking it.[18] MSM is a beneficial form of organic sulfur, a naturally occurring nutrient found in every living organism. In its purest form, this naturally occurring mineral is white crystals. MSM is a beneficial dietary supplement with a toxicity rating equivalent to water—and the lowest levels of toxicity in biology.

When taken in accordance with instructions on the bottle, you can take it safely with other medications, although I always recommend that you consult a doctor before you take anything in addition to prescription medications. It is best to start with the lowest dose and build up. The lowest recommended beneficial amount of 1,500 milligrams per day, in two or three doses. However, some people take as much as 10,000 milligrams for the specific treatment of arthritis. When I'm busy, especially in the midst of a hectic travel schedule, I use MSM in capsule form. I also like to buy it in its purest, white powder form and mix it with vitamin C. The two work great together, and the combination tastes much better. It can take anywhere from two weeks to a few months to start seeing the effects; your body needs time to get used to it. If you take it first thing in the morning, it will be easier to get into the habit.

Vitamins C and E

These power twin supplements can give your face a lift without a face-lift! How? In a nutshell, they significantly improve skin's health by countering the damaging effects of sun exposure. Whether we're sun worshippers or not, we are all exposed to its rays. Simply leaving the house without sunscreen can cause skin to age prematurely and become dry and wrinkled. Even worse, prolonged sun exposure can lead to skin cancer. Yet your skin needs vitamins C and E desperately—every day. So what should you do? To give your skin robust treatments of vitamins C and E from the inside out, eat foods that are extra rich in these vitamins.

Foods that are rich in vitamin C include citrus fruits, such as oranges, grapefruits, and lemons; red and green bell peppers; broccoli; cauliflower; and dark leafy greens such as spinach, kale, and mustard greens. You can also beautify your skin by taking vitamin C supplements of between 500 and 1,000 milligrams per day.

Foods that are rich in vitamin E include sunflower seeds; almonds; spinach; Swiss chard; turnip, mustard, and collard greens; papaya; asparagus; and bell peppers.

Vitamin A

This vitamin is also essential for a skin-care regimen. If you don't have enough vitamin A, your skin looks dry and flaky rather than young and healthy. Vitamin A maintains and repairs skin tissue, so adding it directly to your skin can result in a significant improvement. You may notice your acne disappearing, wrinkles smoothing, and psoriasis lessening, all because of a skin-care cream rich in vitamin A. An acne-free, wrinkle-free, rash-free face is truly beautiful.

Vitamin B

Vitamin B complex may be the most important vitamin for your skin. Biotin, found in B vitamins, is a nutrient that forms the basis of skin, nail, and hair cells. Without enough biotin, your skin will lack radiance. Be sure to get your biotin by eating foods such as oatmeal and bananas, and applying biotin directly on your skin in a cream or lotion. The results: Your skin will transform, shimmering with a healthy glow. It will retain moisture, stay smooth, and look younger—all in less than a week!

Vitamin K

This supplement is also a big blessing. Nothing looks less healthy than dark, puffy, under-eye circles. To eliminate dark circles under your eyes and reveal beautiful, glowing skin, try using a vitamin K cream or supplement.

Naturally Beautiful Teeth

While in Indonesia on a speaking engagement, I suddenly got struck by a vicious toothache. It was so bad that I suffered through several sleepless nights. I finally went online and discovered natural remedies for toothaches and an abscessed tooth. One site suggested a quick cure of chewing on a clove of garlic. This amazingly worked! I felt fine for the rest of the trip and maintained my sanity. Garlic is a natural antibiotic, killing bacteria and infections, and in most cases works as good as a painkiller.

This experience gave me the determination to learn more about natural ways to cure tooth problems—ways that don't call for toxic chemicals such as fluoride and glycerin or invasive dental surgeries. Having healthy strong teeth not only gives you a great smile and helps you look younger longer, but also "recent studies link oral infections with diabetes, heart disease, stroke, and premature, low-weight births."[19] And there are natural ways to make those pearly whites sparkle without all the toxic overload on your body.

Dr. Weston Price, one of the greatest pioneers in the field of tooth cures, showed how to restore dental health without surgery or chemicals. Dr. Price visited many different indigenous people groups around the world who showed remarkable tooth quality in the early 1900s. Instead of rates of 50 to 95 percent tooth decay like people in modern society, certain peoples exhibited anywhere from 0 to 5 percent! What were these people doing differently? Can their habits or results be emulated? Yes, they can!

The modern way to supposedly protect teeth from decay and cavities is to brush and floss daily. Ironically, this has not seemed to stem the increase in dental problems over the past century. In and of themselves, brushing and flossing are not wrong. Yet they do not cure the problem. If brushing, flossing, massive fluoridation campaigns, and dental surgery were effective in preventing tooth decay, it would not get worse over time as it has. Most ancient people never knew about such things as brushing and flossing.

Notice the difference and the degeneration with the modern diet in the teeth, facial structure, and dental arches in the lower set of photos, compared to the first set. Switzerland's modernized districts show rampant tooth decay. The girl in the second set of photos is older, and the one to the right is younger. They use white bread and sweets liberally. The two children below have badly formed dental arches with crowding of the teeth. This deformity is not due to heredity.

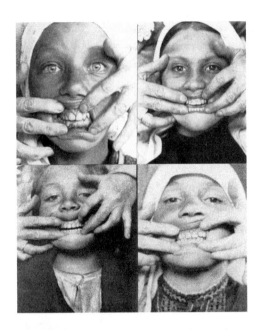

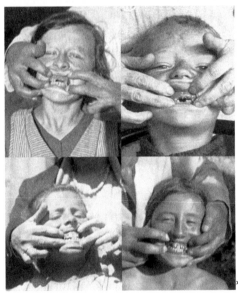

One of the problems with brushing is that most of the toothpaste recommended today contains fluoride. Fluoride is the smallest negative particle and destroys enzyme molecules at very low concentrations. Though marketed as dental protection, fluoride destroys eighty-three enzymes in the body. X-ray studies have revealed the mechanism and process by which it destroys these enzymes.[20] Fluoride breaks up the hydrogen bonds that keep your mouth and teeth intact. It is a nerve poison that causes cavities and unleashes positive hydrogen bonds in enzymes and proteins. Fluoride also detaches the gum tissues, forming deep pockets measuring anywhere from one to eight millimeters.

Clean your teeth naturally

To see your teeth go from natural to super natural health, first stop using all toothpastes, gels, and rinses that contain fluoride and glycerin. "To avoid fluoride is to prevent more than 114 ailments," says Dr. Gerald Judd, a long-time chemistry professor and industry researcher. "These 114 medical side effects extend all the way from cancers down to headaches caused by 1 ppm (parts per million) fluoride in the water. Thirteen of these side effects are proven by a double blind study on 60 patients by 12 physicians, 1 pharmacist and 1 attorney."[21] Even the most "natural" toothpastes contain glycerin, which coats the teeth and prevents re-enameling.

Here are my recommendations for natural cleaning options in place of regular toothpaste:

► Tooth soap (see www.toothsoap.com)

► Making your own with all or some of these ingredients:

2 Tbsps. unprocessed raw coconut oil (also swishing this for a minute a day will help clean and pull out junk from your teeth)
¼ tsp. tea tree oil
¼ tsp. baking soda

2 Tbsps. Extra-virgin olive oil

¼ tsp. spearmint or peppermint oil

Pinch unprocessed sea salt or Himalayan salt

¼ tsp. eucalyptus oil

¼ tsp. food-grade hydrogen peroxide

Put in food processor or blender and blend together. Place a small amount on your toothbrush and use to brush regularly.

Eat your way to healthy teeth and gums

A diet centered around raw grass-fed dairy products, including raw organic eggs, raw milk, raw cheese, raw cream, and butter is paramount for healthy teeth.[22] Some of you may be totally opposed to the idea of any dairy—especially if you follow a vegan diet. I understand your reasoning. The problem is not milk itself but all the processing it goes through. Raw and organic milk and raw cheese contain live enzymes and other raw nutrients needed to reverse the decay process in teeth and help to re-mineralize the enamel, but pasteurization destroys these enzymes. This diminishes the vitamin content and destroys the B_{12} and B_6 vitamins. With the milk's proteins altered and its beneficial bacteria killed, it is no longer a natural food. Instead it has turned into a highly processed junk food that many rightfully claim causes allergies, heart disease, colic in infants, growth problems among children, osteoporosis, arthritis, and even cancer—and increases tooth decay.

If you are a vegan, you can still opt out of eating meat, but increasing raw dairy intake will make a huge difference!

In addition to raw dairy, other special foods include:

▶ Organs of sea animals, and uncooked or slightly cooked wild fish (sashimi, salmon, and tuna, rare or seared).

► Bone broths, such as fish stew broth, is very mineral-
izing for teeth. Bone broths make a good stock that
you can use as a base for a soup or to flavor other
dishes. Fish parts need only boil for about an hour,
while you may simmer other types of stock for a
whole day.

The Creator did not design your teeth to decay the way they do
in the modern world. Our teeth can rebuild themselves and cover
themselves over with a hard and glassy layer—if we give ourselves
the right kind of nutrition. You can minimize tooth decay and even
prevent it entirely—even healing it once a cavity has formed—if you
make the healthy food and hygiene choices.[23]

This combination of beautifying super foods and natural vitamins will reduce photodamage from the sun's rays; smooth wrinkles; keep skin moist and enrich its texture; strengthen nails; give
you fuller, shinier hair; and brighten your smile, without burdening
your body with the many toxins found in popular cosmetics and
beauty products, keeping you healthy, glowing, and simply amazing
for many years to come.

•Chapter 7•

FOODS, SUPPLEMENTS, AND ACTIVITIES THAT REVERSE AGING

Bless the LORD, O my soul, and forget not all His benefits...who satisfies your mouth with good things, so that your youth is renewed like the eagle's.[1]

—King David

O
NE OF THE least publicized subjects is the brain and how it affects everything else in your body. The brain is the control center of everything. Once you learn how to feed and utilize this control center, you can literally start to see drastic changes beyond any diet and begin to experience age reversal! Once you are able to get a handle on brain food, you can greatly control your weight and a host of other conditions, avoiding things like dementia and Alzheimer's disease and reversing the aging process.

Lest you think this isn't important, consider the story released by a scientific publication in the fall of 2012. It explored evidence that Alzheimer's is primarily a metabolic disease, with a poor diet a possible indicator of this degenerative condition. The future forecast is bleak as well, with the thirty-five million Alzheimer's sufferers worldwide projected to reach one hundred million by 2050. Commenting on the long-established links between Alzheimer's and type 2 diabetes—as well as obesity—*Popular Science* contributor Clay Dillow wrote of these findings: "This isn't hard fact or scientific principle just yet, but the evidence is mounting, further reinforcing something that we all know is intrinsically true: you really are what you eat."[2]

Don't let this forecast discourage you, though. The good news is this: the Creator designed our body to re-create itself. Every month your skin renews itself. Every five days you get a new stomach lining. Every three months your skeleton is re-created. Ninety-eight percent of the atoms in your body re-create themselves every year. Even brain cells that cause you to think helped create carbon, nitrogen, and hydrogen. Those same substances were not there a year ago, as well as the raw material that creates your DNA (deoxyribonucleic acid), which is the fundamental building block for your entire genetic makeup. It is renewed every six weeks.[3]

Aging first occurs in the brain. As you age, certain chemicals in your body diminish, which sends a death code to other parts of the body. If you can revitalize these brain chemicals to the levels of your younger years, you can slow down and even reverse the aging process! For example, when a woman's ovaries start to wither, they send a death code to the rest of the body to start aging at an accelerated pace. When you bring the ovaries back to their normal state, it starts to "resurrect" other body parts, regenerating your body to its more youthful state. It all starts with brain health.

The idea is to first discover what part of your body is aging the fastest. Once you repair one part of the body through brain health, the other parts heal and reverse—even before you start working on them.

Brain Power

The brain is the control center and transmits signals to your body. As you age, these signals slow down unless you purposely "wake them up." You can break the death code in your body by resurrecting and enhancing certain brain functions. The brain uses four key chemicals to control the aging process: dopamine, acetylcholine, serotonin, and GABA.

Dopamine

Dopamine is a neurotransmitter released by nerve cells to send signals to other nerve cells. First of all, this vital organic chemical controls your brain's voltage. This determines your metabolism, which determines your weight, ability to process food, and level of consciousness and alertness. Dopamine also affects your brain's power, ability to process information, movement, and emotional response—in other words, almost every area of your body. Low dopamine is one of the fastest age accelerators, sending a signal to the rest of your body to start slowing down and aging. As one example of the problems stemming from low dopamine, people with Parkinson's disease have very low dopamine levels. And there are other impacts:

- ► **Cardiovascular effects:** Low dopamine also puts strain on the heart, making it work harder than normal. This lack of dopamine increases blood pressure and fatigue, causing weight gain. If left unchecked, low dopamine can lead to a clogging of your vascular and blood vessels and possibly lead to a stroke.

- ► **Immune system:** Low dopamine can affect your immune system, starting with the weight gain that often follows when levels are low. Excess fat due to low dopamine hinders your body's ability to fight off viruses and bacteria, which leads to sickness. Obesity speeds up every type of cancer in every organ of your body.

- ► **Menopause/andropause:** Women who are heavier or too thin due to lower dopamine levels can see accelerated onset of menopause. Andropause, the male form of menopause, occurs in men who are overweight due to low levels of dopamine; this leads to low testosterone, low libido, and sexual dysfunction. Loss of testosterone results as muscle turns to fat, first in the abdomen area, and then the rest of the body. For both men and women it also can also be characterized by depression and low energy—like puberty in reverse. Hormone loss is a major age accelerator.

If you can control your dopamine levels and keep your weight down, it can take ten to fifteen years off your age. Things that deplete dopamine levels are stress, poor nutrition, poor sleep, antidepressants, and drug use, as well as alcohol, caffeine, and excess sugar.

So, what do you do to increase your dopamine levels?

- ► **Exercise:** This immediately increases dopamine levels, which in turn increases your desire to exercise and your body's energy. The more you exercise, the more you cause age reversal. Your body and hormones start to think it is young again, reversing the death cycle signals. Just thirty minutes of exercise a day will increase dopamine levels and start to reverse the aging process.[4] Exercise will also reduce cortisol and stress, thus strengthening the immune system, and increase circulation to the skin by cleansing the pores through perspiration. Exercise increases muscle-fat ratio, increases bone density—reducing risk of injury—and helps sexual dysfunction by increasing blood flow to the organs. The way you see things and act is the way the body responds. Make sure you are doing different types of daily exercise of at least thirty minutes, such as cardiovascular (walking or running whether on a treadmill or outdoors), aerobic exercise, weights, bicycling, swimming, racquetball, tennis, rebounding, or team sports that include physical activity.

▶ **Supplements and food:** Supplements that will help increase dopamine include tyrosine, grape seed or pine bark, and gingko biloba, along with vitamin C and E and other antioxidants. They help increase dopamine as well as blood flow and energy, focus, and impulse control. Foods that increase dopamine are almonds, avocados, bananas, raw dairy products, lima beans, pumpkin seeds, and sesame seeds. *Avoid* sugar, refined foods, saturated fats, and cholesterol-laden foods, which interfere with proper brain function and can cause low dopamine levels.

Acetylcholine

Acetylcholine increases blood flow to the brain, which improves memory, concentration, and cognition. It governs brain speed, determining how quickly the electrical signals are processed. When you lack acetylcholine, your brain speed slows down, which leads to cognitive mental disorders. When you increase your brain speed by increasing acetylcholine, you will experience improved memory, attention span, IQ, and even behavioral patterns. Low acetylcholine can lead to dementia, Alzheimer's disease, and learning disorders. Your brain starts to dry up when acetylcholine is lacking.[5]

Acetylcholine controls and maintains hydration. Your brain and body start to dehydrate once you are low in this hormone, which regulates your immune system. Then your bones start to lose calcium as your brain tells your bones and cartilage to provide moisture, leading to bone loss, osteoporosis, and arthritis. To avoid all this, boost your brainpower by keeping your acetylcholine production up. It will reverse this process of degeneration. That is why people with Alzheimer's and osteoporosis are usually frail—moisture loss in their brain leads to bone, cartilage, and muscle loss to compensate.

Here are some supplements you should start taking to boost acetylcholine:

1. Acetyl L-carnitine: This boosts acetylcholine, prevents loss of brain cells, slows rate of cognitive deterioration, provides cells with energy, and provides cells with brain health. It is also great for converting fat to energy.

2. Also consider choline, DMAE, fish oils (omega-3), CLA (conjugated linoleic acid), gotu kola, and gingko biloba. (As with all supplements, there are precautions that you must be aware of and acknowledge. Gingko is a blood-thinning agent; if you are on any other blood-thinning agents, such as aspirin or warfarin, then do not take it before consulting a physician. This statement is true for any supplements—check with your health care provider or physician before taking.

In addition, you need to change your diet. If your brain is drying up and you start craving fats, there is a good reason—dehydration. If you start eating healthy fats and other foods to boost your system with choline, you will begin to add back the necessary moisture and hydration to your brain. Some of my favorite foods that contain choline are avocados, raw goat cheese, cucumber, zucchini, lettuce, poached eggs, and asparagus.

You also need spices to boost your brain speed. Some of these include turmeric, sage, mint, black pepper, basil, lemon rosemary, cayenne, and curry (curcumin), which you can add to your food. India has very low amounts of dementia and Alzheimer's disease, which many believe is the result of the high spice content of Indian foods. Studies have shown that dementia and Alzheimer's caused by amyloid plaques formed in the brain have diminished and/or disappeared when humans consume large amounts of curry. In experiments on mice, these plaques also vanished.[6]

Serotonin

In the central nervous system serotonin plays an important role in the regulation of body temperature, mood, sleep, vomiting, sexuality, and appetite. Low levels of serotonin have been associated with several disorders. The notable ones include clinical depression, migraine headaches, irritable bowel syndrome, tinnitus, fibromyalgia, bipolar disorder, and anxiety disorders. Lack of serotonin makes you feel irritable, depressed, and unhappy. Lack of sleep is often associated with low serotonin levels.

One of the fastest ways to increase serotonin is to get more sleep. When you sleep peacefully and long enough (at least seven hours), you wake up feeling refreshed. Many negative emotions often diminish with a good night's sleep. During deep sleep serotonin levels increase, helping to replenish and renew various parts of the body. Have you ever felt totally hopeless and frustrated—and then took a nap or woke up the next day after a long sleep, and the issue that seemed like a mountain had turned into a molehill? This is what higher serotonin levels and sleep can do.

Also, the creative side of your brain is activated when you rest and sleep more. When you are overworked and don't get adequate sleep, this shuts down your creativity, awareness, joy, and peace of mind, which affects your personality. Lack of sleep also increases phobias, fears, and nightmares. Lack of sleep is a major age accelerator. It can weaken the immune system and cause bone loss, skin dehydration, poor circulation, decline in memory and mental awareness, depression, and other complications. Those who sleep better and know how to rest or meditate can tap into creativity, new ideas, and a spiritual state much faster than those who try to get by with little rest. Basically a good night's sleep is like pushing "reset" on your computer when it goes haywire.

In his book *Younger You*, Dr. Eric Braverman—an expert on brain chemistry—says that it takes at least seven hours of daily sleep to boost serotonin levels.[7] Less than forty-nine hours a week will accelerate the aging process![8] Some basic things to help you sleep are avoiding caffeine (not just coffee; countless drinks and other substances contain it), especially in the evening, and avoiding electrical input at night, whether the TV, computer, video games, or smartphones. Instead, read a good book or listen to calming music right before you go to sleep. Avoid naps during the day, as this will keep you up later at night.

You can also take natural supplements like melatonin, tryptophan, vitamin B_6, fish oils, magnesium, and vitamin B_3. (Talk to your health expert or physician about these and any other supplements or advanced treatments.) Some natural foods that help to increase serotonin levels are oatmeal, blueberries, poached eggs, and cottage cheese.

Herbs and spices that boost serotonin are:

- ► Black pepper: aids in epilepsy, sinusitis, and digestion

- ► Cayenne pepper: helps with neuropathy, pain, headaches, and rheumatoid pain

- ► Thyme: controls spasms, respiratory problems, and fungal infections

- ► Turmeric: protects liver and is a natural body cleanser

► Basil: helps lower stress

► Peppermint: helps relieve fatigue and tension

► Borage: reduces inflammation

► Nutmeg: helps with psychotropic properties and alleviates gastrointestinal problems

► Sage: helps relieve fear, paranoia, and delusions

GABA

GABA is a chemical in the brain that causes you to relax, reduces anxiety and stress, and increases alertness, which is why some call it the "peacemaker" chemical. GABA keeps all the other neurotransmitters and hormones in check. People who are GABA-deficient can become irritable and unfocused, experience chronic anxiety, and have difficulty handling the day-to-day stresses of life. Symptoms can also include headaches, palpitations, heart disorders, low sex drive, and hypertension.

Though there are prescription medications that can help the GABA receptors, unfriendly side effects can often accompany them. The best, safest way to go from natural to super natural health and naturally boost your mood is the natural healthy way with diet, natural supplements, and spices.

The aforementioned Dr. Braverman in his book *The Edge Effect: Achieve Total Health and Longevity With the Balanced Brain Advantage* explains, "GABA is also involved in the production of endorphins, brain chemicals that create a feeling of well-being known as 'runner's high.' Endorphins are produced in the brain during physical movement, such as stretching or even sexual intercourse."[9] As endorphins are released, you begin to feel a sense of calm—often referred to as the "Endorphin Effect."[10]

Among the many foods that increase GABA levels are almonds, tree nuts, broccoli, bananas, lentils, brown rice, spinach, oranges and other citrus fruits, halibut, rice bran, whole grains, and walnuts. A supplement that helps boost GABA levels is L-theanine, which calms nerves and increases mental clarity. This amino acid is also found in green tea, which is an excellent way to start the day instead of with coffee.

GABA has a slightly sedative effect, which is great when taking it before going to bed.

Other Beneficial Substances

Marvelous melatonin

Melatonin is also helpful in regard to sleep. All our hormone levels, including melatonin, start to decline as early as our twenties. With less and less of it in our system as we age, we don't sleep soundly. Melatonin has a relatively low toxicity risk for most adults, although children and pregnant women need to consult with their doctor before taking it because it is not clear how it interacts with other hormones.[11] (Actress Suzanne Somers takes a whopping 20 milligrams a night and claims to sleep better than ever.[12]) In addition to the effects of aging, normal cycles of melatonin production are altered due to such factors as medications and light exposure at night.

While the long-term health effects of disrupted melatonin secretion are not yet fully known, some scientists have suggested that years of working nights could lead to adverse effects—even cancer.[13] Fortunately, melatonin supplements can safely and effectively restore balance to the body's circadian rhythm of this important hormone. They can help you enjoy a restful night's sleep and keep your biological clock ticking throughout a long, healthy life span.

Resveratrol: the antiaging supplement

Resveratrol has the power to slow down aging, prevent cancer and infections, and even protect your nerves against breaking down. Needless to say, this is an excellent supplement for people who are aging and who are suffering from different health disorders that cannot be cured by simply taking expensive prescription drugs that are riddled with side effects.

When it comes to slowing down aging, resveratrol's power stems from the fact that it can activate a class of longevity genes found in the body that are known as sirtuins. It has numerous health benefits and antiaging potential. In addition, according to researchers and doctors, resveratrol is the answer to the "French paradox" mystery—namely, that despite indulging in foods and dishes that contain three times more saturated fat than the typical American diet, French people enjoy lower occurrences and deaths related to cardiovascular problems. And it's all thanks to the red wine (an integral part of the French diet) that contains high doses of resveratrol. Resveratrol may help to activate sirtuins, which reduce cellular decay while imparting greater self-rejuvenating power to your cells. Many scientists suggest that this type of gene may exist in all forms of living organisms and that the benefits they bring can be likened to calorie-restricted diets—enhancing cellular respiration and boosting your body's metabolism.[14]

Resveratrol also slows down cellular decay, reduces cell death, restricts the multiplication of abnormal cells, and gives your body more power to repair itself at the cellular level. All of these and more are important enhancers of longevity. Resveratrol capsules can typically be found at your local health food store or at www.sedonanaturals.com or www.jumpstartthebook.com.

The antiaging benefits of HGH

HGH (human growth hormone) is an endocrine hormone produced by the anterior portion of the pituitary gland. Our body's natural production of HGH, made up of 191 amino acids, decreases as we age. On average it declines 14 percent per decade.[15] Humans normally produce about 500 micrograms of HGH daily at age twenty. By age forty production is only 40 percent of that, or 200 micrograms. Double your age again to eighty, and daily production falls to 25 micrograms or less.[16]

Virtually every system in the human body is in some way dependent on HGH for proper functioning. So, thanks to steadily declining production after adolescence, many of the effects of aging become quite evident. Yet clinical evidence and recent medical research demonstrate that replacing human growth hormone in adults who are deficient in it can significantly eliminate these symptoms. This helps reverse the biological effects of aging, reduce body fat, increase lean muscle mass, strengthen the heart, and improve sexual performance. No other substance known to medical science has proven to continually deter and reverse the process of aging. In many cases, with one year of continual HGH therapy you can reasonably expect to reverse 10 to 20 years of age decline.[17]

Among the many benefits of HGH are:

▶ Abdominal fat reduction: Growth hormone promotes the action of insulin. When we use or increase HGH, it directs the action of insulin toward putting sugar into the cardiac muscle and nerve cells rather than into fat cells. By getting rid of abdominal fat, you can induce greater insulin sensitivity. Greater insulin sensitivity can help prevent, and in some cases reverse, Type 2 adult-onset diabetes.

▶ Increased leanness: After just six months of HGH use, patients see an average reduction of 14 percent in body fat; after one year, an average increase of 9 percent in lean muscle mass.[18]

▶ Improved sex drive: Whether male or female, a decline in libido is directly related to age-related declines in HGH and testosterone levels. A clinical study of approximately three hundred aging adults showed that HGH and/or testosterone replacement therapy improved sexual potency and frequency in 75 percent of the men studied. Both men and women who were interviewed stated that there was improvement in sexual function with HGH replacement therapy.[19]

► Fewer wrinkles: Growth hormone helps with the promotion of type-2 collagen, which adds elasticity to the skin.

► Joint healing: HGH has an anabolic effect on soft tissue—tendons, cartilage, other connective tissue, etc. Because of stronger connective tissue, old injuries can repair at an accelerated rate and with more strength.[20]

► Improved metabolic cascade: When we age without rejuvenation, the efficiency of our overall endocrine system—thyroid, pancreas, adrenal cortical, and hypothalamic pituitary axis (HPA)—tires and wears down. In addition to this problem, a degenerative metabolic cascade takes place within the body as it produces fewer hormones and related "messengers" that relay signals from the surface of cells to the interior. Receptor sites also start to lag, and some switch off, or in menopause disappear.

Treatment guidelines

HGH has a potent anabolic effect (synthesizing protein and building tissue), which can cause an increase in the number of cells and enlargement of muscle cells. Restoring, retuning, and maintaining youthful hormone levels help to jump-start tired, worn receptors. Because HGH precursors rejuvenate on a cellular level through cell division, the overall effect of systemic endocrine rejuvenation has a long-lasting list of benefits.

However, it is essential that you follow doctor-administered protocols and with the help of the physician's assistant to monitor therapies. Proper and timely dosage administration, along with nutritional guidance, adds synergy and leads to gratifying results. If you decide to take HGH, it is essential that you take the most natural form of bio-identical (all-natural), high-quality HGH. Consult your physician or an antiaging specialist to locate the best source.

Depending on your age and level of HGH, you may want to start with supplements, exercises, and other natural methods such as limiting food intake before bed, eating low-glycemic meals with high-quality protein, and low-glycemic fruit such as apples, figs, berries, peaches, apricots, and grapefruit to boost growth hormones naturally. If done properly, fasting is highly effective in raising HGH levels. Tests conducted on lab mice show that regular caloric restriction actually prolongs their life span, compared to those that eat all that they want.[21] Fasting puts you in survival mode and induces the body to release HGH to give it added strength to ride out the induced "stress" of fasting. Fasting for twenty-four hours every week or two is a good practice. It helps the body detoxify, cleanses the bowels, and rests the body.

While fasting is also known to increase HGH, this is one technique that should be used sparingly. If you have a history or risk of anorexia or bulimia, you should not fast, since this can trigger the problem.

Boosting HGH naturally

Besides medical treatments, there are ways to boost your HGH levels naturally:

> ▶ Get more sleep. Although Dr. Braverman suggests seven hours, I believe it is better to get at least eight. "Not getting enough sleep regularly can lower the amount of growth hormone your body produces daily," says Walter Thompson, PhD, director of the

Center for Sports Medicine, Science and Technology at Georgia State University in Atlanta.[22] Even though sleep won't necessarily increase the amount of growth hormone your body secretes, constantly burning your midnight oil can suppress how efficiently your body distributes growth hormone during the course of the day. Keeping normal sleeping habits may let you tap into a more consistent amount that sleep-deprived bones never get a chance to utilize. Sleep is when the highest levels of fat burning and muscle recovery occur, so make it a priority.

▶ Follow smarter eating habits: Focus on eating six or seven smaller meals a day instead of three or four larger ones. Also, eating larger meals with a high glycemic index—such carb-rich foods as white bread, white rice, and bagels—forces the body to release a higher amount of insulin into your system to help with digestion. This causes your body to store body fat at the same time it inhibits or slows the amount of growth hormone released throughout your bloodstream. One way to avoid this is to consume other low-sugar foods that will prevent and slow down the release of insulin. When the anterior pituitary gland is able to function at optimal levels, it speeds up the amount of growth hormone released and pumped into your system. This can be achieved by training right, eating right, sleeping right, and keeping stress to a minimum.

▶ Pre-workout food: Food researchers have discovered that consuming a protein-and-carbohydrate-rich meal two hours prior to working out and another meal immediately afterward elicited a significant increase within the bloodstream in both growth hormone and testosterone. To demonstrate the opposite effects, "researchers at UCLA found that subjects who exercised with partially digested food in their stomachs experienced up to a 54 percent decrease in the production of growth hormone. Subjects who ate strictly carbohydrates prior to a workout experienced a lower production of growth hormone by up to 24 percent."[23]

▶ Get the most from your training. A recent study in the *Journal of Applied Physiology* found that the frequency and amount of growth hormone the body secretes is relative to the intensity of your workout. Subjects who exercised at a higher intensity experienced greater and more frequent releases of growth hormone afterwards.[24] To get the maximum amount of growth hormone released from training and fitness exercises, make sure that the duration and intensity of your regimen is high enough to generate a response. A good standard to follow is keeping your workouts focused on short-burst, high-intensity, anaerobic stretching exercises and maintaining a pace that lasts at least twenty to thirty minutes. Sprinting hills, swimming, interval cycling, cardio-boxing, and other exercises that cause you to be completely out of breath will also achieve this result. Research shows that intense anaerobic exercise like weight lifting can increase HGH levels by as much as 500 percent.[25] Try also conducting intense, full-body muscle exercises, such as push-ups, pull-ups, and squats. These exercises encourage the body's neuroendocrine response, which also promotes HGH release.

Other Steps

Taking supplements

A study done in 1980 showed that taking the amino acid glycine immediately before working out can mildly stimulate the release of growth hormone—but only when taken as a supplement.[26] If you try to achieve the same effect by consuming such glycine-rich foods such as poultry or milk prior to exercise, this will only inhibit growth hormone by causing you to exercise on a full stomach. In addition, the glycine doesn't get absorbed in the same way.

Being introduced into the body in the presence of additional amino acids forces the glycine to compete for transport across the blood-brain barrier, diminishing its effect on the growth hormone levels. The only way glycine can cause a reaction is when taken in isolated supplement form, preferably on an empty stomach. This speeds up absorption and prevents outside interference from other amino acids.

Don't pig out before bed

Never eat a large meal within two hours of going to sleep. The reasoning ties into avoiding the same insulin surges you want to prevent during the day before a workout, but this abstention is especially important before bedtime. The body releases the greatest amount of growth hormone during the first two hours of sleep. Having excess insulin within the system after a large meal suppresses this higher output of growth hormone, preventing your body from taking advantages of it as you rest.

Nighttime also seems to be the best time to take additional supplements to increase the flow of growth hormone. UCLA researchers have found that taking the amino acids arginine and ornithine together on an empty stomach right before bedtime can boost growth hormone levels significantly (depending on dosage).[27]

Also, the sleep aid 5-hydroxy tryptophan—a safer derivative of tryptophan—also helps the brain release growth hormone.[28]

God created our bodies to heal themselves and regenerate new cells, skin, hair, teeth, and nails over and over again. But how we provide our bodies with the right building blocks to do this successfully makes all the difference. So don't delay in fueling your body with the nutrition and activities I've outlined here. All you have to lose is a decade off your age!

PART 3

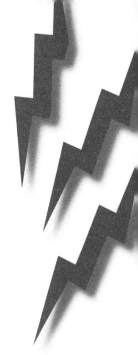

MIND OVER MATTER

• Chapter 8 •

AS A MAN THINKS...

Nothing can stop the man with the right mental attitude from achieving his goal; nothing on earth can help the man with the wrong mental attitude.[1]
—President Thomas Jefferson

JUST AS YOU are what you eat, you are also what you think. The way you see yourself is who you will become. Every action starts with a thought. Once your thoughts start to change about yourself and life, your life starts to change. Because actions are the results of thoughts, to see change you need to allow your thoughts to be conditioned in a way that will bring you maximum results in every area of life. You need to take control of your thoughts and not allow any random, uncontrolled imaginations to dominate your thoughts. Just as raw food has an energy force, thoughts are so powerful that they release energy—good or bad—depending on your thoughts.

When you experience a strange dream, like someone chasing you and trying to hurt you, your heart beats faster. You wake up feeling exhausted, as if this nightmare really happened. Your mind treated it as fact. When you watch an intense, heart-stopping, action-filled movie, your mind sends the same signals to your body as if you drove a car in one of the high-speed chase scenes. This causes reactions in your stress levels, heart rate, and other physical indicators. Your body does not differentiate between whether what you are seeing is reality or simply a movie or a dream. As you see the images in your mind or on a screen, your body reacts positively or negatively.

Thoughts have creative abilities. If you dwell on them consistently, they start to manifest into reality. The more you think and focus on a particular thing, the more it will become a reality.

When you start to think about something negative—for example, how you will pay your bills, if you might get evicted from your home, or if you will lose your job—your body starts to release toxins into your bloodstream. This affects your heart rate, arteries, energy, and immune system, just to name a few.

Thoughts of anger, rejection, fear, or bitterness all produce negative physical effects. Not only does this rob you of peace and joy, but it also releases dangerous toxins into your body. Just thinking about certain negative events or possibilities can adversely affect your life. Negative thoughts start to spiral you downward. You devote so much energy to these thoughts that you are then worn out and depleted. Drained, you cannot think and act on thoughts that build you up and drive you to achievement and super natural health.

When you often dwell on negative thoughts, people can pick up on that and sense something negative. When your presence drains those around you, they tend to distance themselves from you. Plus, when you live in a constant state of fear and anxiety, you are primarily hurting yourself by depleting your immune system. Such people will get sick much faster than those who don't live and think this way. Start to think on things that are helpful, exciting, positive, and energizing!

Visualization

When you see yourself achieving great health and joy, thinking the best of people and generally dwelling on positive thoughts, it helps rejuvenate your cells, which improves your health! If you start to see yourself in great internal and external shape, your mind will send a signal to your body that will help you to achieve this or any other goal.

When I started to really get serious about health years ago, not only was my body affected, but also my outlook on life changed. Suddenly a new faith came upon me that literally anything was possible and all the dreams God gave me were ready to come to pass. A newfound joy and ability to immediately start tackling those new dreams and vision started to erupt. I woke up totally hyped up, excited, and full of a new strength, energy, and joy, which resulted in everything I started to create and do, including lifelong dreams being accomplished in a short span of time. The wind was in my sail, and God and His angels seemed to be on my side like never before, opening up new doors, opportunities, and connections. For example, one of the things I did was to start to write this book that I knew I was destined to write; I also created a company called Sedona Naturals, giving people access to many of these needed supplements and products. I also started to go on radio and TV seemingly all at the same time, when something began to click in my spirit, body, and mind—all being renewed at the same time.

Just as there are laws of gravity and laws of flying (airplanes), there are also laws that affect the natural and spiritual realms. As wise King Solomon put it in Proverbs 23:7, "For as he [a man] thinks in his heart, so is he." Thinking you are more than able to attain super natural health or weight loss will cause you to achieve it. If you think there is "no way" that this can happen, that is what you will get. Most sicknesses originate with wrong thinking, leading to wrong actions about food choices or emotional patterns, which leads to sickness.

You need to take full control of what you allow to enter your mind. If it is a negative thought, quickly replace it with a positive thought. Meditate on the time that someone told you they loved you, or the birth of a child, an honor in school or at work, or other positive experiences from your life. You have to take negative thoughts captive and then send them packing. After all, everything you see around you started as a thought in someone's mind and then came into manifested reality. You are what you think about and how you see yourself.

Maintaining a positive outlook extends beyond yourself too. People respond to external stimuli, so when others can visualize optimistic outcomes in present circumstances, it inspires them to push forward in their own lives. The "winners" among us are those who see possibilities, offer hope, and help us push beyond ordinary limits. They have overcome the innate human condition, which is to grumble, complain, and reason that things will never get better. While I realize that in recent years the economic downturn has seriously affected the circumstances of millions of people, that doesn't mean conditions will never improve.

Nor does a pessimistic outlook necessarily reflect reality. In an essay for *Time* magazine, Charles Kenny—author of *Getting Better: Why Global Development Is Succeeding and How We Can Improve the World Even More*—noted that falling mortality amid rising world population runs counter to the gloomy idea of increased population producing a global breakdown. Espoused in the late 1700s by economist Thomas Malthus, the pessimistic "Malthusian trap" predicted that increased population meant increased poverty, famine, and war as people scrapped for limited resources. Instead, Kenny wrote that the spread of wealth reduced global poverty by more than half since 1990; after two dozen wars in 1984, by 2008 that number had declined to five.

"The spread of global democracy, better health, more education, less violence—it all adds up to a much better world," Kenny said. "And that suggests the biggest new idea of all: it's time to abandon our usual pessimism about the state of the planet and the course of history. We've got many challenges to overcome, but it might be a good idea to adopt a bit of youthful optimism when it comes to confronting them. After all, we appear to be making pretty good progress."[2]

Overcoming Past Thoughts

How do you rid yourself of negative thoughts that have been in your mind since youthful days? Many people were conditioned from childhood to dwell on negative thoughts because of the influence of parents, teachers, other authority figures, and classmates. Maybe your father told you that you would never succeed or did not show the love you needed. You might have been bullied at school. Because such negative experiences might have been etched into your mind at a tender age, it affected all your decisions or indecisions—affecting future relationships and your adult life. Oftentimes as adults we discover hidden anger or resentments against those we blame for our present circumstances.

To start changing, you have to first take charge of your life and not let someone else dictate who you were created to be. The most powerful force in the world is forgiveness. Forgive the person or persons who hurt you in the past, which will set you free to move on and create a new future. As bad as it was at the time, continuing to hold on to what someone said or did will only limit you and continue to lead down a self-destructive path. If you hold on to resentment, then they win and you become the "loser" that people predicted you would become. However, if you forgive and let go of the past, you win and prove to be the opposite of the curse of gloomy words someone spoke over your life. Once you forgive them, it will feel like a million pounds of weight lifted off of you—freeing you from a prison of defeat and opening the cell door to a new life of limitless possibilities.

Recently I read a reflection on ways to forgive those who have wronged you by author Marelisa Fabrega. She mentioned listening to an interview with former President Bill Clinton in which he recalled the time he asked famed South African leader Nelson Mandela how he had forgiven those who had unjustly deprived him of his freedom for twenty-seven years: "Mandela answered, 'I didn't want to be in prison anymore.' When you refuse to let go of hurts from your past, you're keeping yourself imprisoned."[3]

Forgiving others may free them too. Even if you don't speak to them personally, the original culprit or culprits may sense a new freedom inside after years of harboring a hidden or subconscious sense of guilt for how they treated you. Try it right now; simply say, "I forgive so-and-so from what they did or said to me." Say it several times to imprint it into your psyche and spirit. If you do this, you will launch a crucial step to super natural health. Indeed, this is the most powerful thing you can ever do! You will notice a new joy and find others attracted to you because of the new sense of love and forgiveness exuding from you.

Personal Practices

Once you have overcome the past, utilize the following practices to propel you toward achievement and fulfillment.

Guilt by association

If you constantly associate with people who put you down or constantly express cynical, critical, and negative views—and don't want to change—then you need to find some new friends. Associating with positive people can propel you toward the successful person you want to become. "Guilt by association" is true. You will take on the positive or negative attributes of those you spend time with.

When you hang around with angry people, you tend to be angrier than before. Others' antagonistic attitudes will slowly but surely creep over you as you tolerate them and stew in their juices. To quote King Solomon again: "Make no friendship with a man given to anger, nor go with a wrathful man, lest you learn his ways and entangle yourself in a snare" (Prov. 22:24–25, ESV).

Focus on the good

You always move toward those things on which you place your focus. Focus on how you will feel when you achieve a particular dream or goal. Once you start to imagine how that will feel, you can tap into the future, experiencing the feelings of joy and satisfaction of a future event before it unfolds. Your mind can't always tell if what you are thinking is in the present or future. It will simply start to cause your body, spirit, and everything else to react *now* according to what you are thinking, whether it be present, future, or past.

This is why you should focus on things that are noble and positive. As the apostle Paul advised, "Finally, brethren, whatsoever things are true, whatsoever things are honest, whatsoever things are just, whatsoever things are pure, whatsoever things are lovely, whatsoever things are of good report; if there be any virtue, and if there be any praise, think on these things" (Phil. 4:8, KJV).

As you focus more attention on your goals and aspirations, your brain will start working overtime to find solutions in your subconscious—even while you sleep. You will also receive help from above. As you attune yourself to the patterns and laws that govern how things function in the invisible spirit world, the Creator will operate in your life. Your mind is like a computer chip that has limited capacity. If you focus your mind on a negative problem and constantly fret over what may happen, your thoughts can get overloaded with fear. Even if a solution was downloaded to you, there would not be any more room in the memory bank of your mind to receive the message. If the message box on your answering machine is full, you cannot receive life-changing messages.

Clear your mind of fear and worry so that you can make room for the solutions that will come to you once you create the proper environment to receive them. Your mind is like a memory card that only contains so much memory. If it is overloaded with worry, stress, and negative input, it will be much harder to receive a fresh download from above.

Desire the best

What you think about often leads to stronger desires. When you couple consistent thinking with desires, they start to manifest into reality. The stronger a desire, the faster you will act on it. Again, it all starts with thoughts. If you have a casual desire for good health but are not motivated enough to act, then your desire needs to increase until it spurs you to action. This needs to take place in the same manner that you strongly desire chocolate chip cookies because of a commercial you keep watching repeatedly. The end result is the same: you act, only in this case it is by running to the store to buy them, making your weight struggles that much worse.

If you start to think thoughts of what you want to achieve or visualize yourself thirty pounds lighter, eventually you will act in accordance with those desires. Again, as I mentioned earlier, thoughts and visuals have an effect on the body, mind, and spirit. At night when you dream, your body and mind do not always know the difference between a present reality and a future scenario. As I mentioned earlier, the same is true when watching a TV show or movie. Even though imaginary, your heart can race during an intense scene. A mental picture in your brain can start working for you or against you. See your future and destiny. Meditate on them consistently, and you will start to attract the necessities, connections, and resources to fulfill your vision.

Speak positive words

The words you speak have an amazing impact on everything you do as well your body. Speech is powerful, so powerful the Bible records the world originating with these words from the Creator: "'Let there be light'; and there was light" (Gen. 1:3). Although invisible to the naked eye, speech and sounds are real objects. If an opera singer can sing at a high enough pitch to break glass, then this force must be a tiny object—like a pebble, only smaller. At high speeds or frequencies it can pierce through other objects.

Scientists call these "sound waves." Sound waves created by speech are so small that if you were to divide the smallest particles and atoms up into some of their smallest forms inside these atoms, at their core you would find a vibrating wave called a quark. These sound waves are embedded in everything on the earth, including rocks, food, trees, and everything ever created. This means that speech was one of the first ingredients that created everything you can see and the invisible things you can't see. This means that these sound waves can be altered and respond to other sound waves or speech.

Pioneering physicist Albert Einstein grasped the power of sound, light, and other forms of energy. His theory of relativity explains it well. In simplified terms, his famed theory, $E = mc^2$, means that E is energy and M is matter or substance. Basically Einstein concluded that energy is real and is considered matter, even though it is invisible to the naked eye. You cannot see electricity itself, but you know it is real when you turn on a light and see it in action. Thoughts and speech release energy. So when you think and speak certain things, you are actually releasing matter or creating things—good or bad.

The Power of Sound Waves

In studies conducted by Japanese researcher Masaru Emoto, water particles and other subatomic particles responded to sounds and words spoken to them.[4] If this is true, then every created thing can—in a sense— hear and respond in some way. While this may sound a bit mystical to some, remember that everything created contained the same core ingredients: sound and light. In some nations such as Canada (where the method is legal) doctors use a procedure called high-intensity focus ultrasound, meaning high-energy sound waves, to destroy cancer cells.[5] Imagine the power of speech against sickness, especially if you use the highest power source—the Creator—when declaring to objects such as disease that they must vanish.

Start to speak the things that you want to see manifested in your life. If you are going for a job, start to say that you are going to have great favor with everyone you meet and that you will be successful. Start to tell your body that it is strong and healthy and that no sickness can survive in such a healthy state. Sometimes I will even say with great joy and humor that my body is so healthy that sickness does not feel comfortable around me and just has to leave. Sound crazy? Quantum physics, science, spiritual giants, and ancient philosophers seem to confirm otherwise. Practice creating your day each morning by speaking what you believe will be created. After connecting to the Creator's power and love, affirm that you will be successful in all that you do, that you are full of energy, and that you will have favor with everyone you meet. This will cause things to shift from the invisible realm to the visible realm and will also take you from natural to super natural health. In large part, your health will be determined by how well you control and bridle your speech to create health and life. As Solomon said in Proverbs, "Death and life are in the power of the tongue, and those who love it will eat its fruit" (Prov. 18:21).

Food Affects Thoughts

When you continually eat unnatural and processed foods, these dead foods that lack natural energy will start to drain you and make you feel less energized. Such sluggish feelings will lead to feeling grouchy, negative thoughts, and negative speech. Eventually, what you eat will affect your thoughts. And your thoughts will affect what you eat. For instance, a lack of an amino acid called tryptophan can lead to depression.[6] Tryptophan is found in raw, high-protein foods such as goji berries, spirulina, chlorella, blue-green algae, maca root, cacao, and other raw foods. Through cooking, tryptophan is destroyed, as it is sensitive to heat. Meats contain this amino acid, but if you eat only cooked meat and potatoes (a bad combination for your digestive system), the amino acid is destroyed. So start to incorporate raw foods into your diet and see the difference it makes in your mental outlook. This will truly be a case of mind over matter!

Another thing that completely disarms your mental power is stress. In the next chapter I will identify key stressors in life that hold us back from overall health and from achieving our dreams and goals. And even more, I will show you how to overcome those stressors, recharge your brain, and get back in the game.

•Chapter 9•

SUPERCHARGED AND STRESS FREE

*Don't worry about anything; instead, pray
about everything. Tell God what you need,
and thank him for all he has done.*[1]

—The apostle Paul,
writing to the Philippian church

S TRESS. IT'S EVERYWHERE. People are stressed mentally,
physically, and emotionally. In one recent survey eight of
ten employed Americans reported feeling stressed out on
the job because of heavier workloads and low pay. Eighty-three percent felt stressed by at least one thing at work, an increase of 10 percent over the previous year.[2] Another survey reported 35 percent
of Americans say their stress increased over the past year. The top
stressors included money (69 percent), work (65 percent), and the
economy (61 percent.) The most stressed were Millennials—people
born between 1980 and 1995. More than half said stress had kept
them awake at night in the previous month, and they have the
highest rate of a diagnosis of depression or anxiety disorders.[3]

This is serious. If not managed and relieved, stress can weaken your immune system, increase weight gain, and cause many sicknesses. Stress is not an illusion, a figment of your imagination, or an unstable emotion; it can be measured. When under stress, your body reacts and changes. This can mean rises in blood pressure, heartbeat, adrenaline production, and breathing, and increased blood and sugar pumped to your fingers and toes.

When someone feels threatened, they go into a "fight-or-flight" mode, usually opting for the latter so they can flee the threat of real or perceived danger. Stress has positive elements (the Creator designed it to help the human system), particularly in life-and-death situations—for example, escaping from a lion in the jungle or a bear in the forest. You are likely more acquainted with the kind that involves an urgent deadline, when the stress factor kicks into gear and you operate at peak performance. Athletes facing a heart-pounding scenario with less than a minute left on the clock rely on stress to help them win. Whether it is winning a game, securing a job, or attaining a goal, stress can put you over the top. Recovery from these temporary situations proves fairly easy.

However, stress was never meant to be an ongoing daily feature of life. This is where it gets dangerous. Ongoing stress is harmful, releasing toxins known as "stress toxins." If not drained away, these toxins can clog up your entire system. Exercise is the fastest way to release stress. When you experience this type of stress on an ongoing basis and don't release it through exercise or deep relaxation, your body gets clogged up with toxins. These harmful substances weaken your immune system, leaving you wide open to stress-related diseases—high blood pressure, cancer, ulcers, heart attacks, diabetes, and much more.

Stress affects not only the body but also the mind. Your mind's memory bank can only handle so much. A perceived threat or the fear of not knowing and imagining the worst possible outcome can create stress for many people. You can get stressed by a perceived problem, such as your boss calling you into his office or someone not returning your call—and failing to connect could cost you your job. However, you can learn soon after that your boss called you in to congratulate you or ask a simple question. Or you quickly see your call returned, with an apology from the caller for misplacing his cell phone.

When you are stressed, your mind is so obsessed and focused on the fear of what *might happen* that you block everything else out. You can neglect your body and get into bad habits of eating and sleeping. Stress can affect your relationships, making you irritable, prone to overreacting, and even paranoid as you imagine that everyone is out to get you. This adds conflict that only multiplies existing stress with additional emotionally based stress. This leads down a slippery road. Unless you take control, you can reach the point of no return.

In its simplest form, stress means living in *fear*. However, most of the time when you fear the worst, magnifying your stress, things turn to be nothing or far less than you expected. Perception makes the difference. One person's positive perception is another person's worst nightmare. The one with the positive outlook stays happier and healthier, and as a result lives a longer, more productive life.

Facing the Perfect Storm

Often a combination of small stresses can lead to an overwhelming sense of hopelessness. Such stressors as your car breaking down, a job layoff, a family member's sickness, and learning your retirement account just lost half its value—all at the same time—can cause "the perfect storm." Yet even in the midst of apparent calamity, remember this: *our perceptions cause our stress.* It's our perception of the event, and not the event itself, that causes our stress. What causes you stress may not even faze me, and vice versa.

What are the most important ways to manage stress?

Exercise vigorously

It is vital that you get regular, vigorous exercise—whatever your doctor advises. Occasionally you are likely to hear someone proclaim that we have such a high rate of stress-related illnesses today because we are facing so much more stress. However, some researchers believe that we aren't dealing with any more stress than our ancestors did.[4] They believe that the high rates of stress-related illness happen because our modern lifestyles don't include the vigorous exercise that earlier generations automatically gained through physical labor. Exercise basically cancels out the effects of stress reactions on our bodies by draining off its toxins.

Relax regularly

Another effective stress management technique is to use deep relaxation, which neutralizes the negative effects of stress. Practice the relaxation response for about twenty minutes a day in a comfortable position. Praying and singing to the Creator works! A good massage and spending time in the sun, similar to a day at the beach, will help you relax and give you a different outlook.

Recognize that attitudes and perceptions play a key role in managing stress

Realize that those dark scenarios you envision means you are probably overreacting. Most of the things you fear the most never happen. Change your perceptions, and anticipate the best instead of expecting the worst. What you believe as fact often comes your way because you can create it by your thoughts. Believe for the best!

Maintain realistic expectations

Many of us create stress by setting our expectations unrealistically high. This is especially true if you are a perfectionist. Plan out bite-sized tasks that you know you can do, and then check them off when finished, which will give you a sense of accomplishment. Do what you can. Write out your plans for the following day the night before. Then, once something has been accomplished, check "done."

Arrange your life so you feel in control

You don't have to be in control of everything. You just need to feel you have some sense of control over your schedule and your lifestyle. Plan how you will start to resolve whatever dilemmas you are facing, and then tackle at least one of those obstacles immediately. If creditors are harassing you daily to pay an outstanding bill, then take control instead of letting them control you. Call them and tell them what you can pay within the next week or two. Then you will gain a sense of control instead of letting stress dictate your daily routine.

Build and maintain a working support network

This is the system that supports you in times of need and makes you aware that you are part of a bigger whole, toward which you have responsibilities. Support networks are particularly important when you are under stress. Remember that one of the problems caused by stress is tunnel vision—an inability to look at alternatives and options. Stress also makes you feel paranoid, as if people are out to "get you" or are purposely being difficult just to aggravate you. Share your perceptions with the important people in your life to see if you are seeing things clearly. Ask them if they see the situation the same way you do. Ask if they have any ideas about what you can do about it.

Spend time with your loved ones

Strong families tend to spend time together often. Unfortunately, when families get stressed out, a natural tendency is for the individuals to go off on their own or to lash out against those closest to them. Don't shoot down your closest allies! One of the healthiest things a family can do when under stress is to purposely spend some time together, go for a walk, or simply get out of the house and away from the TV or computer in order to do something fun outdoors.

Balance your commitment to your children, job, loved ones, and yourself

Either too much or too little emphasis on ourselves is unhealthy. We need to constantly search for that happy middle ground for both ourselves and our families.

Only you can determine the amount of stress that is healthy for you. The amount of stress you need to operate effectively, at your very best, is very personal. No matter what the setting, decide how much stress you can manage. Then monitor it so that you don't take on less or more than is healthy and productive.

Electromagnetic Stress

Staying indoors too much can cause stress, especially when you are in a place that has any electromagnetic waves—namely, those generated by such devices as cell phones, computers, appliances, ovens, airports with heavy electromagnetic interference from control towers, smart electric meters, or microwave generators. Stress from these waves are caused by electromagnetic radiation called EMFs (electromagnetic frequencies), which are caused by magnetic fields. Appliances and cooking have EMFs, but they dissipate the farther you are from the kitchen. But high-powered sources of EMF, such as powerful transmission towers and lines, travel up to hundreds of feet right through walls. The same applies when you are around many devices that are plugged into your wall.

EMF is invisible—yet so damaging and harmful—and has been shown to cause cancer. As far back as 1982 the *New England Journal of Medicine* reported that utility workers had double the incidence of leukemia compared to men in other occupations.[5] Prior to that, two doctors at a Veteran's Administration hospital in Syracuse,

New York, showed that mice exposed to low-frequency EMFs from power lines gave birth to stunted babies.[6] And detailed examinations of childhood mortality records in metropolitan Denver by two University of Colorado researchers correlated long-term exposure to EMFs with a higher incidence of cancer.[7]

Other studies have focused specifically on the suspected connection between EMF exposure and cancer, including reports showing a major connection with EMFs and the incidence of leukemia, lymphoma, and cancer of the nervous system in children.[8] The Environmental Protection Agency has tried to warn the public, but the powers that be realize the huge financial losses to utility and other industries if the entire infrastructure of the modern world had to be changed.

To avoid exposure, try not to sleep right next to electrical gadgets, especially those with higher EMFs that plug into a wall outlet. Keep appliances a good distance away from your body—on the other side of the room or in another room, as well as cell phones, computers, and other devices.

Cell Phone Dangers

Given the ubiquitous presence of smartphones on college campuses, offices, and buses or subway systems worldwide, my warning about cell phones may sound extreme. Yet they are a leading hazard. Cell phones emit levels of radio frequency (RF) in the same range as electromagnetic-radiation-causing microwaves. Even the industry admits that cell phones are not safe. In one of its publications Motorola says: "It is well known that high levels of RF can produce biological damage through heating effects..."[9] The user's guide for one of the company's phones says: "A few animal studies, however, have suggested that low levels of RF could accelerate the development of cancer in laboratory animals. In one study, mice genetically altered to be predisposed to developing one type of cancer developed twice as many such cancers when they were exposed to RF energy compared to controls."[10]

It goes on to explain similar studies on humans. The manual says of this human impact: "When tumors did exist in certain locations, however, they were more likely to be on the side of the head where the mobile phone was used.... An association was found between mobile phone use and one rare type of glioma, neuroepithellomatous tumors."[11] Maybe it isn't surprising that I have noticed that when I hold a cell phone for too long on one side of my head, it can cause sharp pains that drain me of my energy!

Cell phones can also interfere with pacemakers. For example, under "Additional Safety Information," the Nokia 6560 User's Guide states: "Pacemaker manufacturers recommend that a minimum separation of 6 in. (15.3 cm) be maintained between a wireless phone and a pacemaker to avoid potential interference with the pacemaker."[12] Most phones used today are many times more powerful than the Nokia model, emitting much more powerful EMFs due to the higher technology of smartphones that can do now what most computers can do.[13] The Nokia User's Guide advises people with pacemakers not to carry the phone in their breast pocket and to hold the phone opposite the pacemaker.[14] If this can occur with pacemakers, I don't want to be a statistic years down the road, when more research can establish stronger links between improper cell phone use and cancer (and other diseases). It's no wonder most hospitals tell people to turn off and not use their cell phones in certain areas where patients are being treated.

Limiting exposure

Cell phones are manageable for short calls but were not designed for extended use. Here are several recommendations to limit your exposure to cell phones:

► Always put the speakerphone on and stand a few feet away. Use a home phone for longer phone calls. A group of researchers in Israel conducted a study to narrow down the type of harm extended cell phone use can inflict on users. They picked a group of twenty-somethings who had used cell phones for an average of 12.5 years and about 30 hours of talk time per month. For the control group the researchers used deaf volunteers, since they virtually never used a cell phone. They compared the saliva of the cell phone users with that of the nonusers. Saliva tests are one of the ways doctors can test for oxidative stress that leads to cell dysfunction, damages DNA, and predetermines the onset of many diseases.

At the conclusion of the study the researchers found that flow, total protein, albumin, and amylase activity were decreased even in the deaf volunteers. This indicated that indeed there was an indication of higher oxidative stress among cell phone users, which may indicate a higher risk for certain cancers.[15]

► Buy a radiation-free headset. Normal headsets send the radiation right into your ear. The radiation emitted from a wireless, radon-free tube headset keeps radiation away from your brain. Even cordless home phones are dangerous since they send radiation to the device. Put the speakerphone on, and keep the phone at least a few feet away when talking instead of putting the phone up to your ear.

► Buy a Biopro Cell Phone Chip for your cell phone and computer. These are chips that you stick to your phone to neutralize the dangers of radiation from electromagnetic frequencies. I always have one on my phone.

► Buy a Q-Link necklace. Worn as a pendant, these devices reduce the harmful effects of EMFs generated by cell phones, computers, and other devices. During frequent airline travels, where I am in the presence of people communicating on wireless devices, air traffic control towers, and other electronic devices, I notice that the Q-Link increases my energy and helps me bounce back quickly after speaking trips. In fact, I have so much more energy it often takes a day or two to adjust. When wearing the Q-Link, world-class athletes have noticed improved mental focus and endurance, giving them a competitive edge.

Other Helpful Suggestions for Becoming Less Stressed

See a chiropractor

Often the stress of an improperly aligned back can add more stress to your life and affect your nervous and immune system. In the past three decades the field of neuroimmunology has published a significant amount of research showing a connection between the nervous system, the immune system, and subluxations of the spine, which refers to its proper structural alignment.[16] A spinal adjustment removes lactic acid and removes stress (so will a good massage.)[17]

Walk barefoot

This is a relatively new trend. Not only will it help relieve stress, but also people who walk barefoot in childhood encounter fewer foot troubles compared to those who always wear slippers, sandals, or shoes. Barefoot enthusiasts have fewer foot deformities, greater flexor strength, and more foot agility, and are able to spread their toes to a greater extent than others. Says one podiatrist, "Toddlers keep their heads up more when they are walking barefoot. The feedback they get from the ground means there is less need to look down, which is what puts them off balance and causes them to fall down."[18] Regardless of the extent to which shoe companies go to create footwear that suits the shape of feet, they can never beat the comfort of walking barefoot. Those who walk with shoes encounter more aches and pains in the body compared with those who do barefoot walking at home.

Benefits of Walking Barefoot

- Barefoot walking helps straighten out the toes. At the same time, when you walk barefoot, it prompts even the lazy muscles of your feet to move. This additional development provides more tone and much stronger foot muscles.

- Another positive effect, which most people are unaware of, is how it helps the leg muscles pump blood back to the heart. This makes it beneficial for those who are suffering from varicose veins.

- It helps relax tired feet and has proven beneficial for people suffering from flat feet—in many cases helping them overcome the problem altogether. Why? *It works the muscles in the feet that are never used.* Some barefoot walkers report better arches forming from walking barefoot. Shoes often protect the feet so much that certain muscles grow lazy from inactivity.

- Walking barefoot in the summer has a cooling effect on the body, especially those who walk on morning grass, leaves, or a piece of log in the garden.

- Traditional exercise enthusiasts (i.e., the martial arts) teach that being barefoot helps you stay more connected and focused.[19] Walking on the ground helps you connect with the earth's natural vibrations, which serve to ground you in the same way as those who walk on the beach. As you walk with your feet bare, you increase your vitality. At the same time, it helps you think clearly and increases your capacity to work.

- Walking barefoot in your garden or at a park will help you feel closer to nature and cause stress to diminish. This will take your mind off everyday tensions, relax your body, rejuvenate your mind, and boost your energy levels.

There are now special, minimalist-type shoes that have been designed to help launch your barefoot walking. However you approach this effort, start slowly and gradually work your way up. At first your feet will get sore quickly, as the muscles are not used to being worked. With most shoes you walk with your heel first, but walking or running barefoot causes you to typically land on the ball of your foot toward the lateral side. Start by walking around the house barefoot or in your yard. Then try walking for maybe half a mile and gradually build up to longer lengths until you can do more. It should cause an overall healing effect. It will connect you with the energy of the earth; diminish stress on your feet, legs, and body; and cause an overall feeling of relaxation and freedom. Go ahead—throw off your restraining shoes!

The Rest Principle

Even the Creator rested on the seventh day. If you work nonstop seven days a week, you will burn out. You need to take a day to completely cut off contact with work, cell phones, computers, and other stress inducers. Originating with the Hebrew language, the word *Shabbat* means a once-a-week sabbatical. Seeing the benefits of sabbaticals have prompted some companies and other organizations to offer several weeks or even months off to long-term employees. While you may not have the opportunity for such an extended break, you can still spend one day a week resting, rejuvenating by talking to the Creator, spending time outdoors, reading, or meditating as you listen to music. That day of rest will cause your other six days to be twice as productive. This is how our Creator made humans to function. Those who rest at least once a week have better physical, mental, and emotional health. So take a day off to be with yourself, your family, nature, and your Creator. You deserve it!

Chapter 10

SUPER NATURAL POWER TO LIVE A **WHOLE** AND **HEALTHY LIFE**

If you can imagine it, you can achieve it. If you can dream it, you can become it.[1]
—Inspirational writer William Arthur Ward

THE INVISIBLE WORLD is more real than we think. In fact, it determines what occurs in our visible world. Recent studies in quantum physics have discovered that subatomic particles change form simply by being observed by humans.[2] As in the case with water particles, when scientists addressed them in a certain way, they would change form. These changes occurred whether these words were angry, filled with love, or connected with other emotions. That everything created on this earth is made up of core subatomic particles, which can be altered by human observation, is simply amazing! Just thinking about certain things immediately causes either a positive or negative effect on your body—whether angry thoughts releasing poisons or happy, loving thoughts releasing healing.

If this is true, then objects in the invisible world change and re-create via simple observation or even our thoughts. By observing something that is in your future and thinking about it, invisible subatomic particles will start to shift, causing things to change from mere potential to reality. In other words, whatever you think about and speak sparks the creative process. When you get a creative idea or inspiration and think about it more intensely, something is already happening. When you start to speak and declare that you will do this, the reality of fulfillment accelerates. Soon after, action follows on your behalf. Before you know it, you "run into" someone or receive a phone call that opens the door to the very thing that started as a download into your brain—a creative thought from the Creator. You become what you think and speak about.

As I started to get into a high place both in my health and with God, everything seemed to just start happening on a faster higher level. For instance, I kept thinking about Australia and how I felt I should speak there since I was passing through Australia on my way to Vanuatu to speak and meet the president and prime minister. I kept thinking about Australia several times a day, and by the third day I received a very big invitation to two major cities in Australia, which was perfect since we were passing through there anyway, and this was really meant to be. When you are connected with the Creator and you think His thoughts at a high enough level or frequency, these thoughts start to materialize into actual substance or reality in our world, because He is the one through which we move and have our being. What He sets in motion will be established in our lives—this goes for our health and our success in life.

The first chapter of Genesis records the reality that the Creator spoke, which led to creation coming into existence. While some treat this as a fairy tale, it makes more sense today than ever, given the scientific language and discoveries to explain how this could be possible.

Your Brain: A Radio Transmitter

Many do not realize that the human brain acts like a radio transmitter, sending out frequencies. Have you ever thought about someone you needed to call for a few days, and suddenly they called you, commenting that they had been thinking of you for the past three days? When the intensity of thought is strong enough, it sends a signal to others' brains. Everything is made of atoms, protons, electrons, and frequencies, including thought and speech.

If an opera singer can release invisible sound waves at a certain pitch strong enough to break glass, so can a strong enough thought create subatomic particles in the form of frequencies. Researchers performed experiments to prove the point that every object contains a certain amount of frequency.[3] I once heard of one experiment where they took a bar of gold and aimed radio frequencies at the gold bar. When they measured the frequency on the gold bar, they discovered that the vibration and frequency of the gold changed when they aimed a radio wave or X-ray at it. Next, they experimented with a person intensely aiming thoughts at a gold bar. They discovered these brain waves caused the vibration and frequency emitting from the gold bar changed in equal measure to the radio frequencies.

Thoughts can send out a weak signal or a strong signal. Have you ever suddenly been hit with a heavy, dark, feeling of sadness and wondered why, since no natural situation existed that would cause you to feel that way? Then shortly afterward you discovered someone was very upset with you and was not only intensely thinking thoughts but also speaking negatively about you? You just discovered the reason. The reverse occurs when you feel a sense of excitement, like something really good is about to happen but you don't know why or what. A few days later you discover that someone made a favorable decision on your behalf. You just experienced receiving the frequency transmitted days before the reality's manifestation.

Our brains transmit energy on different frequencies. What you think about also affects physical matter. A story I once heard brings this revelation home: A doctor mixed up the results of two different patients. One patient had full-blown cancer and only had three months to live. The other patient's tests showed he was cancer free. When the second man learned that he supposedly had cancer and only had three months to live, immediately his brain sent strong signals that indeed he had cancer. He thought about it day and night. His emotions reflected this belief, as did his actions—he planned his funeral. Within three months he developed terminal cancer and died. The brain of the man with cancer but mistakenly thought he didn't sent signals of healing to his body. He started to dream again of all the things in life he wanted to accomplish. He canceled his funeral plans, gave thanks for his healing, and became more grateful about his life. When checked again three months later, his cancer had gone into remission and he was cancer free. Both patients' brains released powerful, intense radio-type frequencies. In turn, they created responses and signals in the body.

Just thinking about something that makes you angry, sad, or depressed can cause your immune system to start shutting down, your heart to beat faster, and your blood to rush to your face, and it can prompt the release of negative toxins into your bloodstream. These toxic thoughts of anger, resentment, bitterness, rejection, and the like will clog up your system. The point is not that you will never experience such thoughts; the difference to your health is how fast you dispose of them. One rule of thumb is to never go to bed in a negative frame of mind. Release these thoughts before going to sleep so they do not flow through your system all through the night. The best way is to simply say aloud: "I release this situation," or "I release and forgive that person." In addition, discipline your mouth not to speak about such feelings. If you continue speaking about them, your words will re-create the situation. As those thoughts start to kick in again, it will re-create the past all over again, producing the same toxic emotions that you experienced originally.

The Power of Prayer

Another interesting concept: if objects and people can pick up thoughts and words, imagine the power of thoughts and words if a person connects to the Creator in meditation or prayer. Then imagine the power of those words compared to someone not connected to a higher power. It seems throughout history that the spoken words of certain people carried much greater power than those of the average person, to where they held audiences spellbound. Some of the most famous people in history had such power when they spoke. It was as if they were backed up by intense thought frequencies—and a powerful spiritual force they received in personal times of reflection or meditation, even during tough times (like famed English Prime Minister Winston Churchill in World War II). These are the same kinds of words and phrases employed today in everyday language by people who recognize the power of thoughts and words. If used correctly, thoughts and words can create situations that did not otherwise exist.

Words That Create

By conceiving your goals and destiny and consistently meditating on them, you create the invisible framework for thoughts to manifest themselves. Once you have done this, it is time to kick your progress into turbo mode! Words spoken with absolute belief, faith, and certainty will bring unity of focus and transform those words into reality. For example, if you casually say, "I will become an A-list actor," but your thoughts and beliefs don't match your words or beliefs, this causes an imbalance and hinders its visible manifestation. Or you might say, "I will lose thirty pounds by this date and be in the best shape possible, and nothing will stop me!" If you speak with conviction and passion while clearly visualizing a thinner, healthier you, then you are going to see it happen. You have incorporated everything about yourself—words, thoughts, passion, and emotions—in unison, at a higher level.

When you speak something that you intend to become reality, what percentage of power exists in those words? Are your mind, body, passion, and focus 100 percent when you speak? Or are you speaking something with just a tenth of thoughts, passion, and intensity? The degree to which your mind, emotions, thoughts, will, passion, and words are congruent at the same level will determine the speed and probability of what you are speaking to take place. Putting the unity of mind, body, will, emotions, and actions behind your words will spark a high level of energy and focus. This means there will not be much that can stop the thing you are aiming for to become reality.

Passion is an integral element of this empowered focus. When you are totally passionate about something that you feel or know you are supposed to do—or become—things start to come your way. Your level of emotion, intensity, and drive is a determining factor in seeing it to reality. You have to want something bad enough to do something about it. Without the internal force of passion, you aren't likely to take the action that will lead to you reaching your vision or destiny. For some people, a diagnosis of cancer from a doctor or some other serious illness serves as a driving force to change their lifestyle. To others it won't be a negative possibility driving them, but a glimpse into the future and how they will feel when they are lighter, thinner, and more energetic. That joy of who they can become sparks their passion and drive!

You can go through all the steps mechanically and still miss the mark if you don't feel this sense of excitement and passion in whatever you undertake to accomplish. If you could do anything in life and money was not an object, what would you do? Start to work toward that desire in life that naturally drives you, and you will accomplish so much more than trying to do things that others expect of you. Their expectations will not necessarily motivate you, which is one reason you should seek to lose weight and get healthier—for yourself. A secret to success is finding your purpose in life, which fuels passion and kicks your outlook into overdrive.

Everything produces itself after its own kind: apple seeds produce apples, orange seeds produce oranges, and bean seeds grow beans. So it has been since the beginning of time. You have natural talents and abilities that you were born with, but the end result of this innate giftedness is not to seek more status, power, or self-glory. Start using those gifts and talents to help others, and you will find a great sense of fulfillment. This will also draw you closer to the Creator. So many people just exist and do not passionately live life to the fullest. They have not tapped into what they are destined to do or realized the fulfillment of their natural talents, gifts, and desires. The world is waiting for their release.

Obstacles to Progress

We often associate a certain goal with pain and suffering. Maybe the last time you went on a diet or tried to jump-start an exercise program, something went wrong and you ended up gaining more weight or hurting yourself at the gym. Then a book like this comes along that can help you change. However, standing in the way are the bad mental and emotional memories of past experiences that block you from taking action. It is like your conscious mind is saying, "Wow, this is great!" But then by the time you have decided to take action, all these fears and other mental blocks associated with this past failure hinder your progress.

Overcoming such obstacles means reprogramming your mind and body. You can do this by starting to associate change with pleasure, such as imagining how good you will feel and look as a "new you," not by what happened the last time you tried. You can also reprogram your mind by reminding yourself of all the sicknesses you will avoid by starting on this new, super natural health lifestyle. The same is true for any change in life you desire. If you can associate with a positive outcome, chances are you will find increased motivation to take action.

When a woman is pregnant or has had lots of pain or complications during earlier childbirth, she may think (or even say), "This is the last time I am going to do this." However, as time goes on and she enjoys the maternal pleasures of raising a baby, she starts to dream again of the joy and pleasure a second child would bring to her, her husband, and her first child. The pain associated with childbirth gets replaced by many more positive memories of the new baby as time goes on. This leads to having the faith to overcome negative programming and focusing on the positives associated with a second child.

What about when someone applies for a new job, or an aspiring actor auditions for a new movie or TV show? Sometimes the fear or perception of past rejection hinders some people from moving on and seeking to accomplish great things. Those who can remove the negative past associations will find the drive to action by a positive vision of the accomplishment and joy they will derive from getting hired for the job or landing that role.

Start to work from the future to the present. Imagine you already have that job, career, published book, or healthy, leaner body. How do you feel now? Have you already arrived at your greatest dream? Or do you see others yet to unfold? As you see, imagine, feel, and enjoy what the future will bring, you are accelerating its existence by tapping into the senses you would feel as if it already occurred! I suggest you consider Paul's words about God, "who gives life to the dead and calls those things which do not exist as though they did" (Rom. 4:17).

You don't have to wait until the future becomes a reality to enjoy the senses and joy of what that will be like. As I mentioned earlier, your body and mind do not know the difference between a future mental image or something occurring today. As you start to see your future and feel the joy of achieving that goal, you will be tapping into your future right now! Then all the other details will start to fall into place. You will get more insights about the next step to take, and before you know it, you will become that which you thought about.

The secret is to first *define your dream or goal* and then have *100 percent passion*—pushing your desire and excitement at full throttle to reach your dream. As you travel on this journey, have a *100 percent belief* that what you are seeing will soon be created. Then take *100 percent action* to reach your goal. Know that it is happening and is out there waiting for you to simply act on it and realize it! Action is where many people stop. You can dream about it and talk about it, but until you finally take action, it will be an unrealized dream.

Start taking a baby step right now toward that dream. It may be a phone call, writing the first page of your book, auditioning for a movie, or starting a business by creating your new business idea's legal structure and name on a site like legalzoom.com—as if you already have a business. The rest will fall into place. As you take your first step, the next step will be clearer as things and the right people and connections will start attracting themselves your way. Bring your future into the present by enjoying, celebrating, and seeing yourself as having already arrived!

Your Highest Source of Power

There are many power sources, but as with everything, high and low levels of power exist. The highest power source would be whatever originally created the power. Creation is extremely powerful. Eating freshly created raw food provides you with a power source.

So does hanging out in the mountains or by the ocean. People meditate or pray to different things, claiming a certain level of power. The Creator who made the creation is the highest power source. The source of all things is the greatest power.

Throughout history some of the most ancient people groups on the earth have known this truth. The Chinese and the first twenty-two emperors worshipped the Creator of heaven and earth. They would offer sacrifices to the Creator, whose name in Chinese is Sheng Ti. In Korean they worshipped the Creator, whose name in Korean is Haniim. The Hawaiians, the Hebrews, Native Americans, and people around the world worshipped the Creator who made everything, seen and unseen. Another common practice is offering a sacrifice of an animal, known as a blood sacrifice. This seems quite strange, even repulsive, to most people in the modern world. Why would blood be so key in accessing the Creator? Well, we know that life is in the blood. If you lose your blood, you will die. The ancient peoples across continents and tribes worldwide always believed that the Creator required and would be pleased by sacrificial blood.

I discovered in researching this that the same story of creation basically spread to the entire world—mankind started off in a physical state close to perfection, and even super human, compared to today. Mankind lost its super human and naturally super natural state when people sinned against the Creator. Instead of loving and worshipping the Creator, mankind started to believe more in the serpent and creation. Humans thought they did not need to love and thank the Creator. In assuming they could be just as good without the Creator's help, they turned away from the Creator's ways.

Once this occurred, the process of death, murder, theft, sickness, toxic living, and other negative influences spread across the world. Ever since then, humankind has attempted to return to the Creator. Blood sacrifice was what the Creator asked the first humans to do to reconnect with the highest power source, according to the most ancient texts around the world, including the ancient Book of Genesis. An innocent animal would have to suffer and die for a guilty person to connect back to the Creator. Blood is symbolic for life on account of man's sin against the Creator.

Changing Sacrifices

The idea of animal sacrifice started to change over the past twenty centuries and now is not as common in numerous cultures (which the animals must like!). However, this is not just because it seems to our natural minds that killing an innocent animal is a sad and cruel practice. Someone changed this dilemma in the human condition. The greatest spiritual being to ever walk the earth changed this entire process. The magi—people who could read and study the stars—learned that something was about to happen. The ultimate super natural Being was about to come on the scene; His original, ancient name is Yeshua.

The magi were stargazers from ethnic tribes in the eastern part of the Middle East. They would follow the exact location where the star would lead them to pay homage to this One who would change everything and reconnect humans back to the Creator. The magi always knew that a Messiah figure would come and reverse the negative consequences of the human condition. Thanks to their knowledge of the stars, now they were able to map out exactly when and where the Messiah would appear.

Their search landed them in the nation of Israel, then under Roman occupation. They told the king at the time why they were there: to find the Messiah who was about to be born. This must have been a pretty big deal. Indeed, they found Yeshua, who had such a profound impact He later split time in half as we know it, from BC to AD. He did this as the only 100 percent pure, nontoxic sinless One. His one act of self-sacrifice formed the connection between humans and the Creator. This one act of allowing Himself to serve as the final sacrifice abolished the need for animal sacrifice practiced by so many cultures waiting for the Messiah. He removed man's guilt and restored peace and harmony in his spirit, soul, mind, and body. Whoever is willing to believe it and tap into this new supernatural life can access the highest power source.

It is recorded that, when Yeshua died, He took on all of humanity's original rebellion, pride, and sin against the Creator. Again, the spiritual law of the cosmos dictated that only a 100 percent, innocent, sinless blood sacrifice could once and for all reverse mankind's toxic, self-destructive patterns. It is also recorded in the annals of history that at Yeshua's death a major earthquake and some type of solar eclipse occurred—and, against all odds, that this Messiah later rose from the dead. The authorities of the time could not handle the fact that the highest power source lived in their midst. They saw Yeshua as a threat. No one else possessed such supernatural, miraculous abilities, or exuded such energy, power, and love. Yeshua could heal, forgive, and even resurrect people who had died. When He resurrected Himself, it proved that there was no other higher source of power that anyone could experience.

This act of love completely removed the wall between humans and the highest power source, the Creator Himself. No longer was an animal blood sacrifice needed for the tribes of the earth to access the Creator; the Messiah had become this eternal sacrifice. Now humans could once again be purified in soul, mind, body, and spirit. They could be redeemed from mankind's toxic, self-destructive nature, reconnecting spiritually and physically with the Creator.

Thanking the Creator

All you have to do now to access the highest power source and experience this incredibly high level of sheer peace in mind, body, soul, and spirit is to tell the Creator that you thank Him for sending Yeshua as a sacrifice so that you could have a direct relationship with Him. Believe that it really happened. Acknowledge that the Creator is the source of all life, and, through Yeshua, you choose to invite Him into your entire being. Tell Him you want to turn away from low-level living and inferior power sources that distract and cut you off from the ultimate true source of love, joy, peace, and health—the Creator of heaven and earth. Invite Him in today!

As you jump-start your journey from natural to super natural health, may you also find a connection with the Creator and experience health—not just in your body and mind, but also in your soul, which will bring you a new joy and life. As you start to...

- ► Change your eating habits and lifestyle

- ► Cleanse your body of harmful toxins and stress

- ► Lose excess weight

...your body will start to transform itself into a beautiful sculpture of youthful, vibrant energy. Your newfound healthy life will start to unfold, opening up dormant creativity and propelling you with a newfound joy to fully discover and achieve your destiny!

I am cheering you on as you make the jump from natural to super natural health!

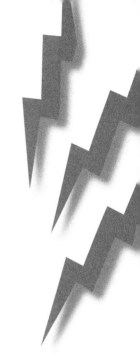

PART 4

TWENTY-ONE-DAY JUMP START TO SUPER NATURAL HEALTH

•Chapter 11•

TWENTY-ONE DAYS TO
SUPERNATURAL HEALTH

*Surely God would not have created such a being as
man, with an ability to grasp the infinite, to exist only
for a day! No, no, man was made for immortality.*[1]

—President Abraham Lincoln

THOUGH MODERN MAN has achieved historic technological breakthroughs that have made life much easier in many respects, in the process we have also lost sight of a great deal of ancient wisdom. In Okinawa, Japan, some residents enjoy the longest life spans on earth, thanks to a diet featuring green and yellow vegetables and much less sugar and rice than other Japanese. Okinawa and other nearby nations report some of the longest life spans in the world. It is common for people to live past the century mark and reach 120 while still exercising, working, and enjoying life.[2] Some health experts also credit their high intake of coral calcium from the ocean, exercise, and peace of mind. The latter stems from living more "connected" to the Creator's original designs for health and rest and limiting the stresses and toxic lifestyles often found in major metropolitan areas.

It just isn't the Okinawans who have benefited from a healthy lifestyle. An ancient Jewish sect called the Essenes broke away from mainstream Judaism and lived in the Israeli desert, away from the city. They lived and ate an extremely healthy diet and regularly performed cleansing techniques like colonics to promote physical and spiritual cleansing. They were some of the healthiest people of their BC era.[3]

If you look at early pictures, Native North Americans looked very slim, muscular, confident, and healthy—until many changed to a Western diet and embraced a more sedentary, indoor-oriented lifestyle. This has resulted in many previously unknown sicknesses and social problems. In the past they were much more connected to nature and the land, but in modern times they have lost much of the ancient wisdom, health, and joy of living. Today the average Native American looks much different physically than their ancestors who lived off of the land. Fortunately, there are an increasing number who are starting on the journey to rediscover the beauty and healing life of eating and living naturally.[4]

The Power of Vegetables

There is an ancient, well-documented story about a Hebrew man named Daniel, who worked for a foreign king in Babylon. The king's servants offered Daniel the best meats, wine, and other delicacies. However, Daniel asked instead if he and his friends could eat a different diet for ten days: raw, healthy vegetables and water, a request that shocked the chief official who had been appointed over them. After the ten days these Hebrews were smarter, stronger, and more vibrant than other residents of the king's palace. Whether or not they followed a long-term vegetarian lifestyle is not mentioned, yet even this short-term experiment proves the different effects healthier food has on the body and mind. It also shows that even in ancient times people recognized the power and benefits of eating high-energy super foods.

Daniel held a high government position and became a spiritual leader by defying the traditional practices of the day. He demonstrated a higher power source than other people in that nation as he prayed solely to the Creator and not the manmade images of the day—which almost cost him his life. In addition to the ten-day fast I just mentioned, later he went on a twenty-one-day fast of only vegetables; at the end of the fast an angel visited him. When you follow a simple diet and live a certain way as part of your daily lifestyle, you can enjoy the same benefits of super natural health.

Like Daniel, it is possible to eat in a certain way for a specific period of time, or even abstain from food for a season, and go from a natural to a super natural state in a very short time. In this super natural state you tend to be much more aware of the spiritual world, with a heighted sense of discernment or intuition. You develop a keen sense of things that prove to be true. Most of all, you seem to access the super natural world much more easily. People groups all over the world have used fasting to do this.

Another ancient prophet named Ezekiel received a divine recipe from the Creator, who told him to live off of this special bread for more than a year, which he did. Today this same bread is available in health food stores and grocery stores across the United States. Instead of flour, Ezekiel bread contains barley, lentils, oats, and wheat. It is understandable why this formula sustained the prophet; this bread contains vital nutrients and super foods.

Many spiritual giants had certain lifestyle differences in their food choices, connections to the outdoors and nature, quiet times to connect to the Creator, and other patterns behind their lives. They seemed driven to a nontoxic life in the natural. Their supernatural, spiritually oriented lifestyle led them toward a healthier, more natural life.

In these next two chapters I am going to share with you my Twenty-One Days to Supernatural Health plan that will jump-start you into achieving supernatural health in every area of your life. You will experience transformation in body, mind, and soul. I will share with you tips on how to optimize natural and spiritual resources to achieve your wellness goals.

Let's get started.

Twenty-One-Day Jump Start
Daily Plan With Recipes and Meal Plan

Upon rising

- ► **Drink 1 cup filtered warm water** with ½ a fresh-squeezed lemon, and some people like to add a sprinkle of cayenne pepper as well (helps boost metabolism). This helps stimulate your liver to release toxins it processed from the night before.

- ► **Go for a morning walk or light exercise/stretching:** Do anything to get your body moving, even just stretching will help jump-start your body first thing in the morning. You may also use a treadmill, but being outdoors is better if possible. The goal is to start somewhere on the first day, and do at least fifteen minutes.

Fifteen-Minute Exercise Routines

Option 1

Stretch your body before doing any exercise.

- Five minutes: do any cardio (If outside, walk, run, or bike. If at home, do jumping jacks, high knees,

front kicks, and run in place.)
- Five minutes: Do lunges or walking lunges.
- Five minutes: 10 push-ups
- Ten sit-ups (or do half sit-ups [crunches] to ease any tension on back)
- Ten squats

Notes: Rest in between if needed, and always have water available to keep hydrated. Do check with your health care professional before starting any exercise program. Feel free to go through this fifteen-minute routine again as you build up your endurance and strength.

Option 2

Ten minutes—aerobic activity:

The goal is for you to do ten minutes of continuous aerobic activity, but what you do is up to you. Most people like to walk, often on the treadmill—it's easy, requires no special training, and it's a comfortable, familiar activity. But others hop on a stationary bike, stair climber, or elliptical machine, or choose to walk outside or in the hallways. Start comfortably, but during the activity move up to a brisk walking pace or effort level—enough to cause noticeable breathing, but still allow you to talk.

One minute—abdominal exercise: fifty half-bent-knee sit-ups

Lay on an exercise mat or the floor with your back flat, your knees bent to about a right angle, and your feet flat on the floor. Pull your chin to your chest and keep it there, and extend your arms and hands, with your fingers pointed toward the tops of your knees. Now slowly lift the shoulders off the mat four to six inches, bringing your hands to your knees, and come back down. That's one; repeat forty-nine more times.

Three minutes—strength moves: beginner

Use dumbbells to do these three moves, selecting the weight so that ten to fifteen repetitions of each exercise is fatiguing.

1. Chest press. Lay with your back flat on the floor and arms extended out to your sides, bent at a right angle at the elbow, hands holding dumbbells. Press the weights up toward the ceiling, fully extending arms, then lower. Do ten to fifteen.

2. Curls. Stand with feet shoulder-width apart, arms straight down at your sides, palms facing the body, holding dumbbell. Bend arm at the elbow, keeping upper arm still but raising the weight to the front of the shoulder. While lifting the weight, rotate so the palm of your hand faces up during the curl; slowly lower weight. Do ten to fifteen on each side, alternating.

3. Shoulder raises. Stand with arms straight down in front of you, palms facing together, holding dumbbells. Keeping elbows slightly bent, raise your arms straight out to your sides, so you look like a large letter "T;" slowly lower weight. Do ten to fifteen repetitions. (Note that you may use substantially less weight for this than for curls or chest presses.)

Three minutes—strength moves: advanced

Eventually try building up to this three-minute routine.

1. Pull-ups. Place hands slightly wider than shoulder width on a pull-up bar, palms facing forward. Pull your chin up to the height of the bar and lower slowly. Ten to fifteen repetitions.

2. Dips. Place hands on parallel bars, with arms straight, supporting your full body weight. Lower until elbows are at a right angle, then press back up. Ten to fifteen repetitions.

3. Chin-ups. Place hands slightly wider than shoulder width on a pull-up bar, palms facing back. Pull your chin up to the height of the bar, and lower slowly. Ten to fifteen repetitions.

One minute—flexibility

1. Side bends. Stand tall, feet shoulder-width apart, hands on hips. Then reach up to the sky with the left hand, bend to the right from the waist, bringing the left hand and arm overhead and reaching to the right. Slowly return to start with hands on hips, then bring right hand up and lean and reach to the left. Continue alternating, reaching and leaning to the opposite side with each hand, with the arm fully extended, for thirty seconds.

2. Sit and reach. Sit upright on the floor with legs straight in front of you. Extend your arms straight, reaching toward your toes, and gently lean forward. You do not have to reach your toes—just stretch to the point that you feel a gentle tension, but no discomfort. Hold for thirty seconds, and then relax. You're done!

1. **Drink a cup of tea:** Drink a cup of organic green tea or rooibos tea (which is naturally decaffeinated) to help your body detox from daily toxins and boost your metabolism for the day.

2. **Make a list of life goals:** While you are having your cup of tea, start by just writing down those things that are important to you, then move into those things that are closer to your heart or you feel passionately about. Don't try to be politically correct, but really search deep into your heart's desires for those things that excite you or that you would love to do even if you weren't paid.

3. **Shower/bathe using your new organic, chemical-free products:** Choose organic natural soaps, body washes, shampoos and conditioners, natural organic face creams, natural toothpastes (and cosmetics as much as possible). This helps keep the chemicals to a minimum for your body to have to detox from, and allows your body to detox those things that are already in your system and get rid of them without the added competition of what is applied on the outside.

A Day in the Life of the Twenty-One-Day Jump Start

Morning

Jump-start smoothies/breakfast (see recipes and plan in chapter 12)

Option 1: The best way is to juice some vegetables and pour the juice into a blender, then add whole fruits and whole vegetables into the blender so that you keep the fiber content. You may also add your other smoothie components such as vitamin C powder and protein powder. Combining juicing with blending gives you the best of both worlds without losing fiber.

Option 2: Eat breakfast using some of the healthy recipes listed under "Breakfast" in chapter 12.

Jump-start new and healthy habits

Assess and really think about any habits that are formed in your life. These twenty-one mornings provide a great opportunity to make changes to form new healthy habits and break old unhealthy ones. Make a list of the good healthy habits in your life, and adjust them to fit as necessary. Also list those habits you want to break free of or change. Remember, if you replace the negative habits with something positive, it only takes approximately twenty-one days to experience lasting transformation!

Lunch (see recipes and plan in chapter 12)

Salads are wonderful to eat for lunch, avoiding heavy carbo-hydrates which tend to make you sleepy and sluggish. Be sure to eat raw live food every day, and salads are great to make sure you are getting the live enzymes your body needs for energy. You may add some protein in the form of organic poultry, small amounts of organic beef, or wild-caught fish to these as well because protein helps provide the building blocks for cells. Choose from the list of salads from the recipe section and change the recipes around for variety.

Afternoon break:

Assess how your day is going. Are there areas that you do not feel peaceful in? Pray and seek peace and wisdom in those areas needed. Make a cup of organic tea and breathe deeply as you seek counsel from the Creator. Stretch your body.

Mid-day snack:

Eat raw live food as it will give you energy. For instance, an organic apple, organic fruit, organic vegetables with healthy dressing for dipping if needed. You can also eat a handful of organic nuts/seeds, organic granola mix as long as you include a raw food with it for the live enzymes.

Snack ideas include:

- ► Ten to fifteen raw almonds
- ► Apple or pear, sliced, with 1 tablespoon raw almond butter
- ► Piece of organic fruit
- ► Carrot, celery, and/or cucumber sticks with hummus
- ► Unsalted gluten-free rice crackers with guacamole or hummus
- ► Kale chips
- ► Smoothie made with organic foods

Dinner (see recipes and plan in chapter 12)

Eat a balanced dinner that includes some protein, organic vegetables, organic whole grains (if not on a gluten-free diet). Try to eat a fresh raw organic salad with dinner along with any cooked foods. Some ideas are:

- ► Grilled, baked, steamed, stir-fried, or rotisserie organic poultry, organic beef, and wild-caught fish
- ► Organic grains such as organic quinoa, organic millet, organic brown rice, organic brown rice pasta, and organic wild rice mix; sprouted grain bread; or Ezekiel bread. You may stir-fry cooked cold millet in place of cooked cold rice in recipes, stir-frying it the same

as rice with excellent results and flavor while adding additional protein. Millet is a gluten-free grain, the least allergenic, and most digestible, and has 15 percent protein, is high in fiber, and is a complete source of protein when combined with legumes. Quinoa is another gluten-free whole grain, with an excellent source of protein with 1 cup of cooked Quinoa providing more than 8 grams of protein alone! It is considered a complete source of protein as it contains all the amino acids required to make up a complete protein.

▶ Salad that contains a lot of green leafy vegetables, as well as bitter greens such as arugula, dandelion greens, spinach, mustard greens, and chicory. These greens help increase the creation and flow of bile for your liver to rid the body of environmental toxins, chemicals, and pesticides.

Evening

Reflection of your day and prayer:

▶ Reflect on your day over a cup of organic tea (rooibos or organic green tea)

▶ What would you do different?

▶ How would you change things for tomorrow?

▶ What new healthy habits do you want to form to go with the new healthy you?

▶ What perceptions do you need to change and replace with new positive ones?

▶ Pray and seek God the Creator for any changes you need help with, forming a relationship and direct communication with Him.

Optional:

Before bedtime, maybe around 9:00 p.m., use an oxygen-based intestinal cleanser dietary supplement on an empty stomach with a glass of water. Drink at least sixty-four ounces of water daily while doing this cleanse to flush out toxins, etc. You can order this supplement from Sedona Naturals at www.sedonanaturals.com. Also consider taking vitamin C each day you are doing the cleanse.

This is considered an effective and safe way to cleanse the colon as it uses oxygen-rich tablets or capsules which are taken orally. They cleanse the intestinal tract by causing the fecal matter in the walls of the colon to melt and be oxidized throughout the upper and lower intestines, which is then easily eliminated. It promotes good bacteria that contribute to a healthy colon.

It cleanses refreshes and detoxifies the digestive tract, and helps restore and maintain regular bowel movements without the worry of negative side effects. Since it is not a laxative, it does not have the negative side effects usually associated with laxatives.

This is an easy way to cleanse your colon on a busy schedule without slowing you down. Follow manufacture directions and check with your health care professional to make sure this is something for you to consider.

Bedtime—10:00 p.m.

Your body needs to go into deep sleep mode during the night with at least seven to eight hours of total rest nightly for adults. This is especially important for your body to function by processing toxins through your liver at night during sleep. Your liver processes toxins while your body is in sleep mode, then as you awaken in the morning it triggers bile to flow into your intestines to carry out the toxins it processed that night out of your body. This is important to allow your body to rid itself of this each day or it will stay in your system/colon and slowly recirculate the toxins in your body causing health issues.

Now that you have an idea for how these next twenty-one days will go for you, let me now give you some delicious recipes and a basic sample on how you can customize meals and activities that best fit your health goals.

Chapter 12

TWENTY-ONE-DAY JUMP START MEAL PLAN AND RECIPES

Week 1 Meal Plan

Day 1

- ▶ **Breakfast:** Very Berry Blush Green Smoothie (with optional protein)

- ▶ **Snack (optional):** 1 organic pear

- ▶ **Lunch:** Chicken Apple Salad with Lemon Dressing

- ▶ **Snack:** Carrots, celery, and/or cucumber sticks with hummus

- ▶ **Dinner:** Chicken With Brown Rice Rigatoni and Vegetables with a small fresh salad

Day 2

- ▶ **Breakfast:** Creamy Green Smoothie (with optional protein)

- ▶ **Snack (optional):** 1 organic apple

- ▶ **Lunch:** Spinach Strawberry Mango Salad (with optional protein)

- ► **Snack:** ½ cup cubed cantaloupe and cucumbers with fresh mint
- ► **Dinner:** Healthy Chicken Wrap with a small fresh salad

Day 3

- ► **Breakfast:** Chocolate Superfood Protein Smoothie
- ► **Snack (optional):** organic strawberries
- ► **Lunch:** Kale With Quinoa Salad
- ► **Snack:** melon with organic grapes
- ► **Dinner:** Broiled Halibut With Corn Salsa and small fresh salad

Day 4

- ► **Breakfast:** Fruits and Vegetables Meal Smoothie
- ► **Snack (optional):** organic peach
- ► **Lunch:** Colorful Brown Rice Salad with gluten-free rice crackers
- ► **Snack:** apple or pear, sliced, with raw almond butter
- ► **Dinner:** Millet Chicken Stir-Fry with a small fresh salad

Day 5

- ► **Breakfast:** Fruits and Greens Smoothie (with optional protein)
- ► **Snack (optional):** organic plum
- ► **Lunch:** Quinoa Salad Delight (may add optional protein)

- ► **Snack:** Ten to fifteen raw organic almonds or nuts of your choice
- ► **Dinner:** Asian Chicken Salad

Day 6

- ► **Breakfast:** Grape and Greens Smoothie (with optional protein)
- ► **Snack (optional):** organic nectarine
- ► **Lunch:** Kale Salad With Grapes (may add protein option of lean poultry)
- ► **Snack:** organic baby carrots with hummus
- ► **Dinner:** Salmon With Spinach Salad

Day 7

- ► **Breakfast:** Berry Greens Protein Smoothie
- ► **Snack (optional):** organic banana
- ► **Lunch:** Tabbouleh Millet or Quinoa
- ► **Snack:** kale chips
- ► **Dinner:** Cilantro Lime Chicken Salad

Repeat this basic format for weeks two and three for a total of twenty-one days, exchanging recipes from the recipe list below for variety.

Recipes and Tips for
the Twenty-One-Day Jump Start Plan

Teas

▶ Green tea or rooibos tea (naturally decaffeinated) or your favorite organic herbal tea

▶ Drink hot or cold

▶ Add lemon, or add almond milk for creaminess

Smoothies and blending tips

▶ A high-powered blender (one that is 1,000 watts or more) works best to make smoothies as it helps release all the nutrients from within the fruits and vegetables, and can process anything frozen with ease.

▶ Freeze seasonal organic fruit to use later in your smoothies until the next season they are available.

▶ To help with any bitterness from your green smoothie, add one to three pitted medjool dates, an extra pear, or additional liquid stevia to taste. Or just simply add more fruit for sweetness.

▶ Smoothie too thick? Add coconut water or filtered water to thin it out.

▶ Add healthy fats to help you absorb the carotenoids found in greens: avocados, virgin organic coconut oil, flax seeds, or chia seeds.

▶ Use for a base: coconut water (naturally contains electrolytes), coconut milk, almond milk, hemp milk, fresh juiced green vegetables, or filtered water.

► Use frozen coconut water ice cubes. Coconut water adds natural sweetness and electrolytes.

► Add super greens powder or protein powder to your smoothie to boost the nutrition.

► Use a wide variety of greens and vegetables in your smoothies, switching them out and rotating them around for optimal health.

► Adding chia seeds is a nice addition to your smoothie (add them at the end). They contain fiber, omega-3, and antioxidants.

Smoothie Recipes

VERY BERRY BLUSH GREEN SMOOTHIE

8 oz. coconut water (or coconut, almond, or hemp milk for
   creaminess)
1 cup organic spinach
1–2 fresh organic bananas
1 cup frozen mixed organic berries with cherries
2 dates (for sweetness)
1 tsp. chlorella
1 tsp. maca

Variation: Vegan Protein Smoothie: Add 1 scoop of raw vegan organic protein powder, organic pea protein powder, or organic hemp protein powder for additional protein.

Blend altogether in blender and enjoy!

CREAMY GREEN SMOOTHIE

2 frozen organic bananas
2 cups coconut, almond, or hemp milk

3–4 large leafs of organic kale

2–3 cups organic spinach

1 tsp. maca powder

1 tsp. chlorella

Variation: Vegan Protein Smoothie: Add 1 scoop of raw vegan organic protein powder, organic pea protein powder, or organic hemp protein powder for additional protein.

Blend all ingredients in blender until smooth!

FRUITS AND GREENS SMOOTHIE

6 oz. coconut water (or coconut, almond, or hemp milk for added creaminess)

1 scoop vitamin C powder (optional)

1 Tbsp. organic coconut oil (optional)

1 organic apple

1–2 organic stalks of celery

½ organic avocado (adds delightful fluffy texture and healthy fat)

Handful organic cilantro leaves (adjust this to preferred taste)

Handful organic frozen mixed berries

Variation: Vegan Protein Smoothie: Add 1 scoop of raw vegan organic protein powder, organic pea protein powder, or organic hemp protein powder for additional protein.

Blend first seven ingredients until smooth, and then add the frozen berries. Blend to desired consistency; add a bit of filtered water if it is too thick. Lastly, add protein powder and blend gently.

BERRY GREENS PROTEIN SMOOTHIE

6 oz. coconut, almond, or hemp milk

Dollop of almond butter, sunflower seed butter, or cashew butter

1 scoop powdered greens (or a handful of organic fresh spinach, with
a bit of organic fresh kale)

¼–½ avocado

Handful organic frozen mixed berries

2 drops liquid stevia if necessary to taste

1 scoop of raw vegan organic protein powder, organic pea protein
powder, or organic hemp protein powder

Blend all the ingredients except the protein powder until smooth. Add the protein powder and blend gently.

CHOCOLATE SUPERFOOD PROTEIN SMOOTHIE

1 cup coconut, almond, or hemp milk

¼ cup goji berries

1 Tbsp. cacao powder

1 Tbsp. maca powder

½–1 cup frozen organic mixed berries

1 fresh or frozen organic banana

1 Tbsp. organic coconut oil

1 scoop of raw vegan organic protein powder, organic pea protein
powder, or organic hemp protein powder

Blend altogether in blender and enjoy!

CHOCOLATE SMOOTHIE

6–8 oz. coconut, almond, or hemp milk

1 organic banana

2 Tbsp. cacao powder

For added protein: Use 1 scoop of raw vegan organic protein powder, organic pea protein powder, or organic hemp protein powder.

Blend altogether until smooth.

SPIRULINA BERRY SMOOTHIE

1 organic banana

2 cups organic blackberries

2 tsp. spirulina

2 tsp. acai juice

Blend all ingredients in blender until smooth, adding more juice to your desired consistency.

TROPICAL SMOOTHIE

1 cup water or coconut water (or coconut, almond, or hemp milk for creaminess)

1 cup pineapple, cubed

1 mango or papaya, sliced

1 banana

2 cups fresh spinach

½ cup frozen blueberries or frozen mixed berries

¼ cup goji berries

Blend altogether in blender, adding spinach last; blend until smooth.

PEACH GREEN SMOOTHIE

6–8 oz. filtered water or coconut water

1 organic peach, chopped or 1 cup organic frozen peach slices

1 organic banana

1 handful organic spinach

1 handful organic kale

½ organic avocado

For added protein: Use 1 scoop of raw vegan organic protein powder, organic pea protein powder, or organic hemp protein powder.

Blend altogether until smooth.

GRAPE AND GREENS SMOOTHIE

6–8 oz. filtered water or coconut water

1 cup organic blueberries, fresh or frozen

2 cups organic red grapes

1 organic pear, sliced

½ organic cucumber, chopped

2 cups organic baby spinach or leafy organic greens, chopped

For added protein: Use 1 scoop of raw vegan organic protein powder, organic pea protein powder, or organic hemp protein powder.

Blend altogether until smooth. Add more or less liquid to desired consistency.

FRUITS AND VEGETABLES MEAL SMOOTHIE

6–8 oz. filtered water or coconut water

1 cup watermelon, cubed

1 cup fresh organic strawberries

1 organic apple, sliced

1 cup frozen organic mixed berries

1 organic tomato

1 organic carrot

1 cup fresh organic spinach, chopped

2 tsp. soaked chia seeds (optional)

Blend altogether in blender until smooth. Add more water if too thick to suit desired consistency.

VEGETABLE AND FRUIT SMOOTHIE

2 cups filtered water or coconut water

1 mango, peeled and pitted

1 medjool date, soaked for 20 minutes

½ organic cucumber

3 oz. organic bok choy, chopped

2 oz. organic beet root greens, chopped

1 organic tomato, chopped

2 tsp. vanilla essence

Place tomato, mango, and date in blender and blend until rough blend. Add the rest of the ingredients and blend on high until smooth.

GREENS AND TROPICAL FRUIT SMOOTHIE

6–8 oz. of filtered water or coconut water

4 leaves organic romaine lettuce or mixed organic lettuce

1 stalk organic celery, chopped

2 fresh organic bananas

1 cup frozen mango, cubed

2 tsp. soaked chia seeds (soak for 10 minutes)

For added protein: Use 1 scoop of raw vegan organic protein powder, organic pea protein powder, or organic hemp protein powder.

Blend bananas and chia seeds with your liquid until a rough blend, then add the rest of the ingredients and blend on high until smooth.

CUCUMBER APPLE SMOOTHIE

6–8 oz. filtered water or coconut water

2 organic apples, chopped

2 medium organic carrots, chopped

½ cucumber, chopped

1 cup organic dandelion greens or mixed organic bitter greens, chopped

Blend altogether into rough blend, adding greens last; blend on high until smooth.

Other Quick and Healthy Breakfast Ideas

- ▶ Two scrambled, poached, or fried organic eggs served with quinoa and organic spinach (or kale or lightly cooked zucchini).

- ▶ A salad of lettuce, sprouts, and hard-boiled organic eggs. Dress up with a mixture of olive oil and lemon juice, salt and pepper to taste.

- ▶ Quinoa with fresh berries, chopped walnuts or pecans, and organic yogurt of your choice on top.

- ▶ Steamed yams, scrambled organic eggs, and organic greens of your choice.

- ▶ Berry smoothies or green smoothies with a slice of organic whole grain, sprouted grain, or gluten-free bread with nut butter.

- ▶ Warm ½ cup cooked millet and add a touch of cinnamon, nutmeg, pure maple syrup or raw honey. Top with fresh fruit, raisins, or nuts.

COTTAGE CHEESE AND FRUIT

1 cup organic mixed berries, fresh or frozen
½ cup organic peaches
½ cup organic grapes
1 cup organic low-fat cottage cheese
Organic granola or nuts for topping

Fill bowl with fruit and top with cottage cheese. Sprinkle with organic granola or nuts.

HOT QUINOA WITH NUTS AND DRIED BERRIES

4 cups water

2 cups organic quinoa

½ cup chopped walnuts

1 tsp. cinnamon

¼ tsp. nutmeg

¼ cup dried cranberries

¼ cup dried blueberries

1 organic apple, chopped

Rice, almond, or coconut milk

Honey or stevia to taste

In a small saucepan bring the water to a low boil. Add the quinoa, walnuts, cinnamon, nutmeg, cranberries, blueberries, and apple; simmer until the water has evaporated.

Top with the milk of your choice and sweeten to taste with pure maple syrup, stevia, or raw honey.

Lunch and Dinner Recipes

Organic cooked chicken, beef, or cooked fresh wild-caught fish can be added to any salad recipe for additional protein.

COLORFUL BROWN RICE SALAD

2 cups cooked organic short-grain brown rice, cooled

1 stalk organic celery, chopped

½ organic zucchini, chopped small (may substitute cucumber)

½ organic red bell pepper, chopped small

1 organic green onion, sliced small

¼ teaspoon organic fresh minced garlic

¼ cup dried cranberries

¼ cup golden raisins

2 Tbsp. organic raw pumpkin seeds

2 Tbsp. organic raw sunflower seeds

2 Tbsp. raw chopped walnuts or pecans

Dash of salt and pepper

Seasonal variation: may add cooked cubed butternut squash for autumn recipe.

Dressing

½ cup organic cold-pressed olive oil

2 Tbsp. organic apple cider vinegar

Stevia to sweeten to taste

Whisk altogether and pour over rice salad mixture until desired moistness. (You may use more or less of this dressing according to preference).

QUINOA SALAD DELIGHT

2 cups cooked organic quinoa, cooled

1 organic cucumber, seeded and chopped small

1 orange, chopped small, or mandarin oranges

¼ cup dried organic cranberries

2 Tbsp. organic raw pumpkin seeds

2 Tbsp. organic raw sunflower seeds

2 Tbsp. chopped pecans

Dash of salt and pepper

Optional: May add 3 oz. cooked organic chicken or turkey

Dressing

> ½ cup organic cold-pressed olive oil
> ¼ cup lemon juice (fresh is best)
> Stevia to sweeten to taste

Whisk altogether and pour over quinoa salad. You may use more or less of this dressing according to preference. Combine all ingredients together and toss with dressing. Serve cold.

MILLET CHICKEN STIR-FRY

> 2 cups cooked organic millet, cooled (cook according to package directions)
> 2 cups cooked organic chicken breast (grilled, baked, stir-fried, or rotisserie)
> 1 cup organic snow peas or sugar snap peas
> 2 organic green onions, chopped
> 1 cup frozen organic peas and carrots, thawed
> 1 organic whole egg, beaten
> 1 clove minced garlic
> ¼ tsp. minced fresh ginger
> 1–2 Tbsp. organic peanut oil or coconut oil for stir-frying
> 2 Tbsp. organic tamari reduced sodium soy sauce or Bragg Liquid Aminos soy sauce, or gluten-free soy sauce of your choice.

Add a little oil to skillet and scramble cook the beaten organic egg; place in a bowl. Next, add the rest of the oil, the vegetables, garlic, and ginger to the skillet; stir-fry these together for five minutes. Add the millet, cooked chicken, scrambled cooked egg, and soy sauce; stir altogether. Stir-fry everything for five to ten minutes until heated through. Serve.

For vegan: omit chicken and egg.

TABBOULEH MILLET OR QUINOA

1 cup cooked and cooled gluten-free organic whole millet, or cooked
    and cooled organic quinoa

1½ cups filtered water

3 diced organic Roma (plum) tomatoes or 1 pint cherry tomatoes,
    halved

½ cup organic cucumber, seeded and diced

¼ cup organic green onions (about 2 onions), finely sliced

½ cup organic Italian parsley, finely chopped

¼ cup fresh-squeezed lemon juice

⅓ cup extra-virgin cold-pressed organic olive oil

Salt and pepper to taste

Place all chopped vegetables in a large bowl. Pour lemon juice and olive oil over vegetables. Add seasonings and cooled millet or quinoa; stir to mix. Refrigerate overnight for full flavor; serve cold.

CHICKEN APPLE SALAD

3–4 oz. cooked organic chicken (grilled, baked, stir-fried, rotisserie)

1 organic apple, chopped

½ stalk organic celery, chopped

Small handful of dried organic cranberries or raisins

Organic romaine lettuce or mixed organic herb lettuce

Toppings of your choice: Organic raw sunflower seeds, organic raw pumpkin seeds, organic raw pecans, walnuts, or nuts/seeds of your liking.

Lemon dressing

1 Tbsp. organic cold-pressed olive oil

2 Tbsp. lemon juice (fresh is best)

Stevia to sweeten to taste
Dash of salt and pepper (optional)

Whisk altogether and pour on salad.

SUPER SKIN COMPLEXION SALAD

Organic lettuce, washed and chopped
Organic cucumber, sliced
Organic celery, sliced
Organic avocado, sliced
Papaya, sliced

Arrange a bed of organic lettuce of your choice in a bowl. Layer cucumber, celery, avocado, and papaya on top. Use as much of each ingredient to suit taste. May use an organic olive oil vinaigrette or a lemon organic olive oil dressing of your choice if desired.

RADIATION-FIGHTING SALAD RECIPE

Organic lettuce, washed and chopped
Organic pear, sliced
Organic avocado, sliced
Organic cilantro
Powdered organic spirulina, sprinkle desired amount on top
Kelp, sprinkle desired amount on top
Miso

Arrange a bed of organic lettuce of your choice in a bowl. Layer the pear, avocado, cilantro, sprinkle powdered spirulina, add desired amount of kelp and miso.

May use an organic olive oil vinaigrette or a healthy dressing of your choice as well.

SPINACH STRAWBERRY MANGO SALAD

2 cups organic arugula or mixed greens, chopped

2 cups organic spinach, lightly chopped

1 cup organic fresh strawberries, sliced

½ mango, peeled and sliced

½ cup sunflower sprouts or sprouts of your choice

¼ cup raw organic almonds, lightly chopped

Add any organic healthy dressing or vinaigrette of your choice if desired. You may also add 6 oz. cooked organic chicken or cooked organic turkey, sliced, for added protein.

PEAR GREEN SALAD WITH MINT

1 head organic romaine lettuce or mixed organic lettuce greens

1 organic ripe avocado, sliced

1–2 Asian pears, sliced

½ organic cucumber, sliced

¼ red onion, sliced fine

1 small bunch of mint leaves, lightly chopped

1 handful raw walnuts or pecans, lightly chopped

Or 1 handful of raw seeds of your choice

Toss altogether. You may use a healthy organic vinaigrette or dressing of your choice. You may also add 6 oz. cooked wild-caught salmon for added protein.

MIXED CABBAGE AND CRANBERRY SALAD

6 cups red and green cabbage mixed or Napa cabbage, thinly sliced

1 small organic green zucchini, sliced thin

1 organic green onion, sliced diagonally

¼ cup fresh organic Italian parsley, chopped

¼ cup dried organic cranberries

½ cup organic almonds or walnuts, coarsely chopped

Place a bed of cabbage in a large bowl and layer the rest of the ingredients on top. Lightly top with your favorite organic balsamic vinaigrette and enjoy!

ASIAN CHICKEN SALAD

2 cooked organic chicken breasts, sliced or shredded

6–8 cups baby bok choy, savoy cabbage, or Napa cabbage, cleaned and sliced thin

1 small bunch organic green onions, sliced diagonally

1 organic carrot, sliced thin

2 stalks organic celery, sliced diagonally

¼ cup organic cilantro, chopped (optional)

½ cup organic almonds, sliced or coarsely chopped

2 Tbsp. sesame seeds (toasted optional)

Asian Dressing

2 Tbsp. organic cold-pressed olive oil

2 Tbsp. soy sauce or gluten-free soy sauce

¼ cup rice vinegar

3 Tbsp. raw organic honey or stevia to sweeten

Salt and pepper to taste

Whisk altogether.

Arrange greens on large platter or bowl. Layer chicken and vegetables, and top with almonds, sesame seeds and Asian Dressing.

FENNEL AND GRAPE TOMATO SALAD

5 large collard greens, cut
1 cup sprouts
½ cucumber, sliced thin
2 Tbsp. fresh fennel
½ avocado, sliced
1 handful grape tomatoes

Dressing

2 Tbsp. fresh lime juice
2 Tbsp. organic cold-pressed olive oil
Agave nectar or stevia to sweeten, if desired
Fresh pepper and salt to taste

Whisk altogether.

Place cut collard greens on platter or in a large bowl and layer the rest of the ingredients, top with dressing.

KALE SALAD WITH GRAPES

1 bunch organic kale, stemmed and sliced thin
1 handful each of red and green organic grapes
1 avocado, sliced
½ cucumber, sliced
1 small bunch sprouts of your choice
1 small handful raw organic sunflower seeds
1 small handful raw organic pumpkin seeds
1 lemon
Cold-pressed olive oil
Sea salt
¼ cup toasted pine nuts

May add organic cooked chicken or turkey for additional protein.

Poppy Seed Dressing

¼ cup organic cold-pressed olive oil

2 Tbsp. organic apple cider vinegar

1 tsp. Dijon mustard

½ shallot, diced

1 Tbsp. poppy seeds

1 tsp. raw organic honey

Pinch of sea salt

Whisk altogether.

Place kale in a large bowl and squeeze the whole lemon over the top, and add approximately 1–2 tablespoons olive oil with a pinch of sea salt. Massage this into the kale until the kale is soft and tender. Layer the rest of your ingredients on top and cover with Poppy Seed Dressing.

KALE WITH QUINOA SALAD

1 cup cooked and cooled organic quinoa

10 organic kale leaves, chopped

3 Tbsp. organic cold-pressed olive oil

2 Tbsp. lemon juice (fresh is best)

1 tsp. Dijon mustard

1 large clove garlic, minced

1 tsp. black pepper

½ tsp. sea salt

1 cup pecans

1 cup dried organic cranberries

¾ cup crumbled feta cheese

Dressing

Olive oil

Lemon juice

Dijon mustard
Garlic
Salt and pepper to taste

Whisk altogether until emulsified.

Place kale in a large bowl. Drizzle dressing over the kale; add cooled quinoa, dried cranberries, pecans, and feta cheese. Toss altogether gently.

CHICKEN WITH BROWN RICE RIGATONI AND VEGETABLES

2 cooked organic chicken breasts, cooled, sliced or shredded
1½ cups cooked and cooled brown rice rigatoni
½ cup cooked and cooled organic broccoli florets
½ cup cooked and cooled organic cauliflower florets
¼ cup chopped sun-dried tomatoes
1 Tbsp. extra-virgin organic cold-pressed olive oil
1 Tbsp. freshly squeezed lemon juice
1 Tbsp. reduced-fat grated Parmesan cheese
10 leaves organic romaine lettuce
2 Tbsp. fat-free organic creamy Caesar dressing

Mix the first five ingredients in a large bowl. In a small bowl mix the next two ingredients, and then toss with the rigatoni mixture. Top the rigatoni mix with Parmesan cheese and serve over romaine lettuce that has been drizzled with the Caesar dressing.

HEALTHY CHICKEN WRAP

1 10½-inch sprouted-grain tortilla
3–6 oz. cooked chicken (may substitute chicken with 2–3 oz. turkey, or 1½ oz. reduced-fat cheese)

2 slices organic avocado

¼ cup canned organic black beans (rinsed and drained)

¼ cup chopped organic lettuce

2 Tbsp. fresh organic salsa

Fill sprouted-grain tortilla with ingredients and enjoy.

BROILED HALIBUT WITH CORN SALSA

5-oz. wild-caught halibut steak seasoned with:

Juice of ½ lemon and freshly ground black pepper and salt to taste

Place halibut on broiler pan four inches from heat and broil ten minutes per inch of thickness or until fish flakes easily. Top with ½ cup organic corn salsa (below).

Serve with ½ cup cooked organic brown rice mixed with ⅓ cup cooked green peas

ORGANIC CORN SALSA

2 cups diced organic ripe tomatoes

2 cups fresh organic corn kernels

12 oz. can organic black beans, rinsed well, drained

4 organic green onions, sliced thin

1 or 2 green jalapeños, seeded, diced fine (may substitute chopped organic green chiles, fresh or canned)

½ bunch organic fresh cilantro, roughly chopped

1 fresh organic lime, juiced

½ organic lemon, juiced

3 Tbsp. organic cold-pressed olive oil

¼ tsp. dried oregano

Salt and fresh ground black pepper to taste

Toss all ingredients in a large glass or stainless steel bowl. Cover and refrigerate for at least 1 hour before serving. May be made up to 8 hours ahead. Toss well before serving.[1]

SALMON WITH SPINACH SALAD

4–6 oz. wild-caught salmon fillets

10 oz. organic baby spinach

1 pint organic grape or cherry tomatoes, halved

¾ cup crumbled fresh goat cheese (3 oz.)

¼ cup pecans

Season salmon with salt and pepper; broil on baking sheet without turning until opaque throughout, about seven to nine minutes. Let cool briefly, and then flake.

Place spinach and tomatoes on serving plates; top with cooked flaked salmon, goat cheese, and pecans. Drizzle with your favorite organic balsamic vinaigrette.

CILANTRO LIME CHICKEN SALAD

4 organic boneless chicken breasts

Marinade

2 Tbsp. fresh organic cilantro leaves, chopped

1 or more garlic clove, minced (more or less to taste)

Zest of 1 lime

2–3 Tbsp. fresh lime juice

¼ cup organic cold-pressed olive oil

1 tsp. sea salt

½ tsp. black pepper

Add the chicken to the cilantro lime marinade and toss to coat; store covered in refrigerator for one hour or more.

Preheat grill and cook chicken until done as the juices come to the top, then turn. Cook until internal temperature is 165 degrees. (May also bake or broil in the oven.)

Serve over a fresh bed of mixed organic lettuce, organic tomatoes, organic avocado, fresh sprigs of organic cilantro, and optional organic corn. May add fresh squeeze of lime on top.

ABOUT THE AUTHOR

DAVID HERZOG IS a nutrition coach, a motivational speaker, life coach and a spiritual help to many. David also works in conjunction with the premier supplement manufacturing and distribution company, Sedona Naturals (www.sedonanaturals .com and www.jumpstartthebook.com) He is also the founder of David Herzog LLC and David Herzog Entertainment LLC. David has given thousands of lectures and television and radio interviews during his speaking tours. He has helped actors, entertainers, presidents, Prime Ministers, vice presidents of nations, and other heads of state across the world, as well as leading business figures and health and sports professionals.

He has visited the White House, and David has also shared his keys to good health and other insights at the United Nations. His work as a motivational speaker (mixed with a lot of comedy), has taken him across North and South America, the Caribbean, Europe, Asia, Australia, New Zealand, South Pacific Islands, Africa, Middle East, India, Sri Lanka, and even native tribes of the world. He loves helping people from every sphere of society achieve their highest potential physically, spiritually and in their careers and callings.

In addition to his exciting speaking schedule, he is involved in acting, comedy, and scriptwriting for movies and television. Currently David is working on several new, cutting-edge books.

Other than his passion for super health, David's hobbies include hiking, surfing, reading, writing, singing, comedy, nature exploration, and travelling the globe to the far-away places and tribes many Westerners have never visited. His favorite hobby is spending time with his family and loved ones and the Creator. He is based in his hometown of Sedona, Arizona, one of the healthiest and most spiritually-oriented places in America.

To contact David or book him on a television or radio show, for an interview or for a seminar please contact:

David Herzog LLC
2675 W. Hwy 89A, #464
Sedona, AZ 86336
E-mail: superhealthdh@aol.com

Websites: www.jumpstartthebook.com,
www.sedonanaturals.com, and
www.davidherzogbook.com

You can order additional copies of *Jump Start!* directly from www.davidherzogbook.com, or call 1-928-282-3969.

GLOSSARY OF TERMS

Acetylcholine: A chemical produced by the body vital for healthy brain function. Acetylcholine improves memory, concentration, and cognition, by increasing blood flow to the brain.

Amino Acids: The building blocks that make up proteins. Humans need twenty different amino acids to function properly. Some are made by the body while others, called essential amino acids, must be obtained from foods.

Antioxidant: Substances, like vitamins A, C, E, and beta-carotene, which protect your body from the damage of oxidation caused by free radicals.

Chlorella: Chlorella is a powerful detoxification aid for heavy metals and other pesticides. Numerous research projects in the U.S. and Europe indicate that chlorella can also aid the body in breaking down persistent hydrocarbon and metallic toxins such as mercury, cadmium and lead, DDT and PCB. And, also strengthen the immune system response.

Colon Therapy/Colon Hydrotherapy/Colonics: Colon therapy uses a series of filtered and temperature regulated water flushes into the colon. These water flushes cleanse and detoxify the lower intestine and aid in the reconstitution of intestinal flora. The purpose of colonics is to balance the body chemistry, eliminate accumulated toxic wastes, and restore proper tissue and organ function.

Detox: Body cleansing or detoxification is an alternative medicine approach which rids the body of "toxins." This is usually in the form of dieting, fasting, consuming exclusively, or avoiding, specific foods—such as fats, carbohydrates, fruits, vegetables, juices, herbs, or water.

Dopamine: Dopamine is a chemical naturally produced in the body. It controls the voltage and power of your brain and its ability to process information.

EMF or Electric and Magnetic Fields: An invisible field of electro-magnetism radiated from sources such as appliances, transmission towers, cell phones, and other electronic devices.

Free Radicals: An atom or molecule with at least one unpaired electron, making it unstable and reactive. When free radicals react with certain chemicals in the body, they may interfere with the ability of cells to function normally. Antioxidants can stabilize free radicals.

GABA (gamma-aminobutyric acid): GABA is a non-protein amino acid that functions as a neurotransmitter. It is the primary inhibitory neurotransmitter in the brain, and serves to cause relaxation, reduce stress, and increase alertness.

HGH (human growth hormone): HGH is an endocrine hormone produced by the anterior portion of the pituitary gland.

Homeopathy: Homeopathy is a medical system that uses minute doses of natural substances—called remedies—to stimulate a person's immune and defense system.

Massage: Massage is the manipulation of the superficial tissues of the human body in order to promote deep relaxation, and release tension. Recent research has proven that massage is therapeutic and can soothe injured muscles, stimulate blood and lymphatic circulation, improve structure and function of the body, increase toxic elimination, and more.

Micronutrients: The name given to vitamins and minerals because your body needs them in small amounts. Micronutrients are vital to your body's ability to process the "macronutrients:" fats, proteins, and carbohydrates. Examples are chromium, zinc, and selenium.

Minerals: Nutrients found in the earth or water and absorbed by plants and animals for proper nutrition. Minerals are the main component of teeth and bones, and help build cells and support nerve impulses, among other things. One example is calcium.

Natural Medicine: Natural medicine or healing is the use of non-invasive and non-pharmaceutical techniques for providing wellness.

Nutrient: A nutrient is any chemical element, chemical compound, or combination of chemical elements and/or chemical compounds that contributes to bodily development or is necessary for life.

Probiotics: Probiotics are live microorganisms thought to be healthy for the host organism. Probiotics are commonly consumed as part of fermented foods with specially added active live cultures; such as in yogurt, soy yogurt, or as dietary supplements.

Serotonin: A chemical produced naturally by the body that aids in feelings of well-being, restfulness, and relaxation.

Spirulina: A microscopic blue-green algae in the shape of a perfect spiral coil, living both in sea and fresh water. It is the one of nature's richest source of vitamins, iron, protein, carbohydrates, micronutrients, and beta carotene.

Supplements: Vitamins, minerals, herbs, or other substances taken orally and meant to correct deficiencies in the diet.

REFERENCES

Good Teeth, Birth to Death, Gerard F. Judd, 1996, http:// gerardjudd.com/affidavit.htm.

"Lymphatic Immune Support," *Well Being Journal,* May/June 2000, www.wellbeingjournal.com.

Managing Nano-Bio-Info-Cogno Innovations: Converging Technologies in Society, page 144, William Sims Bainbridge, Mihail C. Roco, 2009.

"Quoting from the Schuphan Study," page 223, *The Sunfood Diet Success System,* David Wolfe, 2000.

Raw Foods Bible, page 74, Craig B. Sommers, 2007. "Ultrasound May Help Regrow Teeth," *ScienceDaily,* June 28, 2006, www .sciencedaily.com/releases/2006/06/060628234304.htm.

RECOMMENDED READING

Cure Tooth Decay, Ramiel Nagel, 2010.

Jumping for Health, Morton Walker, 2005.

Nutrition and Physical Degeneration, Weston A. Price, 2008.

Rebounding to Better Health, Linda Brooks, 1997.

Younger You, Eric Braverman, 2008.

The Maker's Diet Revolution, Jordan Rubin, 2013.

NOTES

Chapter 1
Are You Fit and Free? It's Time to Take Stock

1. Positive Life Quotes, http://positivelifequotes.info/tag/what-you
   -get-by-achieving-your-goals-is-not-as-important-as-what-you
   -become-by-achieving-your-goals-henry-david-thoreau/ (accessed
   August 27, 2013).
2. Centers for Disease Control and Prevention, "Obesity and Overweight," http://www.cdc.gov/nchs/fastats/overwt.htm (accessed
   August 26, 2013).
3. Centers for Disease Control and Prevention, "Childhood Obesity Facts," http://www.cdc.gov/healthyyouth/obesity/facts.htm
   (accessed August 26, 2013).
4. World Health Organization, "Obesity and Overweight," World
   Health Organization, http://www.who.int/mediacentre/factsheets/
   fs311/en/ (accessed August 26, 2013).

Chapter 2
Understanding Nature's Energy Stores

1. Jean Anthelme Brillat-Savarin, "Aphorisms of the Professor," in
   The Physiology of Taste, M. F. K. Fisher, trans. (New York: The
   Heritage Press, 1949).
2. WakeUp-World.com, "Kirlian Photography Demonstrates
   Organic Uncooked Food Have Stronger Energy Fields," http://

wakeup-world.com/2012/01/19/kirlian-photography-demonstrates
-organic-uncooked-food-have-stronger-energy-fields/ (accessed
August 27, 2013).

3. Danny K. Asami, Yun-Jeong Hong, Diane M. Barrett, and Alyson
E. Mitchell, "Comparison of the Total Phenolic and Ascorbic Acid
Content of Freeze-Dried and Air-Dried Marionberry, Strawberry,
and Corn Grown Using Conventional, Organic, and Sustainable
Agricultural Practices," *Journal of Agricultural and Food Chemistry* 51, no. 5 (February 26, 2003): 1237–1241.

Chapter 3
Jump-Start Your Health With a Cleanse

1. Everything Essential, "Cleansing or Detoxification," http://www
.everythingessential.me/HealthConcerns/Detoxification.html
#page=page-1 (accessed August 27, 2013).

2. Melanie Rud, "Colonics: Are They a Waste of Time?", Health.com,
August 3, 2010, http://www.health.com/health/article/
0,,20429816,00.html (accessed August 27, 2013).

3. Mehmet Oz, "High-Tech Ways to Extend Your Life," Oprah.com,
http://www.oprah.com/health/Life-Extension-Technology-and
-Tissue-Regeneration/6 (accessed September 6, 2013).

4. As referenced in Heather Hudak, "Tips to Boost Your Immune
System," *Hudak Holistic Health* (blog), September 15, 2010, http://
hudakholistichealth.blogspot.com/2010/09/tips-to-boost-your
-lymphatic-system.html (accessed August 28, 2013).

5. Morton Walker, *Jumping for Health* (N.p.: KE Publishing,
2005), as quoted in Scott E. Miners, "Bouncing for Health,"
WellBeingJournal.com, http://www.wellbeingjournal.com/
bouncing-for-health/ (accessed August 28, 2013).

6. Linda Brooks, *Rebounding to Better Health*, rev. ed. (Greensboro,
NC: Vitally Yours Press, 2008).

Chapter 4
Eat Your Way to a Healthy Weight

1. Elizabeth Berg, *The Day I Ate Whatever I Wanted: And Other Small Acts of Liberation* (New York: Random House, 2008), 137.

2. Robert Lustig, *Fat Chance* (New York: Hudson Street Press, 2012), 15.

3. Edward Howell, *Enzyme Nutrition* (N.p.: Avery Publishing Company, 1995).

4. Mark Hyman, "How Diet Soda Makes You Fat (and Other Food and Diet Industry Secrets), *Huffington Post*, March 7, 2013, http://www.huffingtonpost.com/dr-mark-hyman/diet-soda-health_b_2698494.html (accessed August 28, 2013).

5. Anne Stein, "Lack of Sleep Contributing to Obesity," *Chicago Tribune*, June 29, 2011, http://articles.chicagotribune.com/2011-06-29/health/sc-health-0629-sleep-20110629_1_sleep-medicine-sleep-disorders-leptin (accessed August 28, 2013).

6. "Caring for a Beneficial Giant: Why Liver Balance Is Important to Health," Maharishi Ayurveda Newsletter Archive, http://www.mapi.com/ayurveda_health_care/newsletters/liver_balance_health.html (accessed August 28, 2013).

Chapter 5
Ultimate Healing Foods

1. GoodReads, "Hippocrates Quotes," http://www.goodreads.com/author/quotes/248774.Hippocrates (accessed August 28, 2013).

2. Sisi Wachtel-Galor, John Yuen, John A. Buswell, and Iris F. F. Benzie, "Chapter 9— Ganoderma Lucidum (Linzhi or Reishi): A Medicinal Mushroom," in *Herbal Medicine: Biomolecular and Clinical Aspects*, 2nd ed. (Boca Raton, FL: CRC Press, 2011), http://www.ncbi.nlm.nih.gov/books/NBK92757/ (accessed September 6, 2013).

3. L. Evets et al., "Means to Normalize the Levels of Immunoglobulin E, Using the Food Supplement Spirulina," Grodenski State Medical

University, Russian Federation Committee of Patents and Trade, Patent (19) RU (11)2005486, January 15, 1994, as referenced in Examiner.com, "Spirulina, the Miracle, Health Aid," September 20, 2010, http://www.examiner.com/article/spirulina-the-miracle -health-aid (accessed August 29, 2013).

4. NutritionalEarth.com, "All About Spirulina," http://www .nutritionalearth.com/Health%20Benefits/spirulina/spirulina.html (accessed September 6, 2013).

5. Naturalways.com, "Spirulina's Nutritional Analysis," http://www .naturalways.com/spirulina-analysis.htm (accessed August 29, 2013).

6. Dani Veracity, "Chlorella as a Powerful Defense Against Cancer," NaturalNews.com, June 14, 2005, http://www.naturalnews.com/ 008527.html (accessed September 6, 2013).

7. D. Campbell-Falck, T. Thomas, T. M. Falck, N. Tutuo, and K. Clem, "The Intravenous Use of Coconut Water," *American Journal of Emergency Medicine* 18, no. 1 (January 2000): 108–111.

8. Natasha Longo, "Get Off Your Thyroid Medication and Start Con- suming Coconut Oil," PreventDisease.com, March 21, 2013, http:// preventdisease.com/news/13/032113_Get-Off-Your-Thyroid -Medication-And-Start-Consuming-Coconut-Oil.shtml (accessed September 6, 2013).

9. Ray Peat, "Coconut Oil," http://raypeat.com/articles/articles/ coconut-oil.shtml (accessed September 6, 2013).

10. ScienceDaily.com, "No Scalpel: Minimally Invasive Breakthrough for Men's Enlarged Prostate Improves Symptoms," March 30, 2011, http://www.sciencedaily.com/releases/2011/03/110329095425.htm (accessed September 6, 2013).

11. American Cancer Society, "What Are the Key Statistics About Prostate Cancer?", Cancer.org, http://www.cancer.org/cancer/ prostatecancer/detailedguide/prostate-cancer-key-statistics (accessed September 13, 2013).

12. J. M. Hodgson, G. F. Watts, D. A. Playford, V. Burke, and K. D. Croft, "Coenzyme Q10 Improves Blood Pressure and Glycaemic Control: A Controlled Trial in Subjects With Type 2 Diabetes," *European Journal of Clinical Nutrition* 56, no. 11 (November 2002): 1137–1142.

13. As reported in William Faloon, "CoQ10 and Cancer: Human Studies Urgently Needed," *Life Extension Magazine*, February 2006, http://www.lef.org/magazine/mag2006/feb2006_awsi_01.htm (accessed August 29, 2013).

14. "Science: The Fleeting Flesh," *Time*, October 11, 1954, excerpt, http://content.time.com/time/magazine/article/0,9171,936455,00 .html (accessed August 29, 2013); Shannon Fowler, "Why New Atoms Aren't a Fountain of Youth," NPR.org, July 14, 2007, http:// www.npr.org/templates/story/story.php?storyId=11893583 (accessed August 29, 2013).

Chapter 6
Nature's Best-Kept Beauty Secrets

1. FamousQuotes.com, http://www.famousquotes.com/show/1028480 (accessed August 29, 2013).

2. Pliny the Elder, *The Natural History* 19.23, http://www.perseus .tufts.edu/hopper/text?doc=Perseus%3Atext%3A1999.02.0137%3 Abook%3D19%3Achapter%3D23 (accessed August 29, 2013).

3. Wisconsin Department of Public Instruction, "Cucumber," http:// fns.dpi.wi.gov/files/fns/pdf/ffvp_fs_cc.pdf (accessed August 29, 2013).

4. N. Otsuki, N. H. Dang, E. Kumagai, S. Iwata, and C. Morimoto, "Aqueous Extract of Carica Papaya Leaves Exhibits Anti-Tumor Activity and Immunomodulatory Effects," *Journal of Ethnopharmacology (Limerick)* 127, no. 3 (February 17, 2010): 760–767.

5. SuperFoodProfiles.com, "How Papaya Enzymes Help Digestion," http://superfoodprofiles.com/papaya-enzymes-digestion (accessed September 6, 2013).

6. As referenced in Heather Hudak, "Calm Your Nerves and Love Your Liver With Celery," *Hudak Holistic Health* (blog), July 7, 2010, http://hudakholistichealth.blogspot.com/2010/07/calm-your -nerves-love-your-liver-with.html (accessed August 29, 2013).

7. FoodReference.com, "Celery Facts and Trivia," http://www .foodreference.com/html/fcelery.html (accessed August 29, 2013).

8. WHFoods.org, "What's New and Beneficial About Celery," http://www.whfoods.com/genpage.php?tname=foodspice&dbid=14 (accessed September 6, 2013).

9. HealthyOurBody.com, "Celery Can Prevent Oily Skin," http://www.healthyourbody.com/2011/06/celery-can-prevent-oily-skin/ (accessed September 6, 2013).

10. RawJuiceCleanseRecipes.com, "Health Benefits of Celery Juice," http://www.rawjuicecleanserecipes.com/health-benefits-of-celery-juice/ (accessed September 6, 2013).

11. Tan Koon Peng, as quoted in Dr. Sircus, "Treatments for Nuclear Contamination," DrSircus.com, http://drsircus.com/world-news/disasters/treatments-nuclear-contamination (accessed September 6, 2013).

12. Kathryn Roethel, "Use Avocados to Make Healthier Desserts," SFGate.com, June 18, 2013, http://www.sfgate.com/health/article/Use-avocados-to-make-healthier-desserts-4608597.php (accessed August 29, 2013).

13. Fabiana Santana, "How Foods Transform You: Eating From the Inside Out," Yahoo! Shine, September 26, 2009, http://shine.yahoo.com/shine-food/how-foods-transform-you-eating-from-the-inside-out-516880.html (accessed September 6, 2013).

14. Jim Healthy, "Onions Are Weight Loss Wonders," MyHealing Kitchen.com, http://myhealingkitchen.com/medical-conditions/weight-loss/weight-loss-healing-foods/low-cal-onions-are-weight-loss-wonders/ (accessed August 29, 2013).

15. A. Lassus, "Colloidal Silicic Acid for Oral and Topical Treatment of Aged Skin, Fragile Hail and Brittle Nails in Females," *Journal of International Medical Research* 21, no. 4 (July–August 1993): 209–215.

16. Nicolas Perricone, "5 Ingredients to Look for in Your Skincare Products," DoctorOz.com, February 3, 2011, http://www.doctoroz.com/videos/5-ingredients-look-your-skincare-products?page=2 (accessed September 6, 2013).

17. O. Re, "2-Dimethylaminoethanol (deanol): A Brief Review of Its Clinical Efficacy and Postulated Mechanism of Action," *Curr Ther Res Clin Exp* 16 (1974): 1238–1242.

18. Stanley W. Jacob, Ronald M. Lawrence, and Martin Zucker, *The Miracle of MSM: The Natural Solution for Pain* (New York: Penguin-Putnam, 1999).

19. Centers for Disease Control and Prevention, "Oral Health: Preventing Cavities, Gum Disease, Tooth Loss, and Oral Cancers—At a Glance, 2011," Chronic Disease Prevention and Health Promotion, http://www.cdc.gov/chronicdisease/resources/publications/aag/doh.htm (accessed August 29, 2013).

20. Gerard Judd, *Good Teeth From Birth to Death* (Glendale, AZ: EMR Labs, LLC, 2001), http://www.rexresearch.com/judd/judd.htm (accessed August 29, 2013).

21. Ibid.

22. Ibid.

23. For more information on natural tooth remedies, I recommend a great book by dental health educator Ramiel Nagel called *Cure Tooth Decay*. I also suggest the writings of Dr. Price, particularly his groundbreaking *Nutrition and Physical Degeneration*.

Chapter 7
Foods, Supplements, and Activities That Reverse Aging

1. Psalm 103:2, 5.

2. Clay Dillow, "Alzheimer's May Be Caused by Poor Diet," *Popular Science,* September 12, 2012, http://www.popsci.com/science/article/2012-09/newest-impact-poor-diet-alzheimers (accessed July 12, 2013).

3. NaturalCuresNotMedicine.com, "How Your Body Rebuilds Itself in Under 365 Days," http://www.naturalcuresnotmedicine.com/2013/02/how-your-body-rebuilds-itself-in-under-a-year.html (accessed September 6, 2013).

4. MedicalDoctorMD.com, "Exercise Is Not Only Good for Your Body," http://www.medicaldoctormd.com/fitness-and-health/exercise-sucks/ (accessed September 6, 2013).

5. Williams.edu, "1A1. Acetylcholine: A Representative Small Molecule Neurotransmitter," http://web.williams.edu/imput/synapse/pages/IA1.htm (accessed September 6, 2013).

6. WHFoods.com, "Turmeric," http://www.whfoods.com/genpage.php?tname=foodspice&dbid=78 (accessed September 6, 2013); NewAmericaMedia.org, "Turmeric Shows Promise in Treatment of Alzheimer's," http://www.vanguardneurologist.com/turmeric-shows-promise-in-treatment-of-alzheimers-2/ (accessed September 6, 2013); *Mirror*, "25 Simple Steps to Help Prevent Alzheimer's," March 2, 2012, http://www.mirror.co.uk/lifestyle/health/25-simple-steps-to-help-prevent-748327 (accessed September 6, 2013).

7. Eric R. Braverman, *Younger You* (New York: McGraw-Hill, 2006), 136.

8. Ibid., 137.

9. Eric R. Braverman, *The Edge Effect: Achieve Total Health and Longevity With the Balanced Brain Advantage* (New York: Sterling Publishing Co., 2004), 12. Viewed at Google Books.

10. Ibid.

11. WebMD.com, "Find a Vitamin or Supplement: Melatonin," http://www.webmd.com/vitamins-supplements/ingredientmono-940-MELATONIN.aspx?activeIngredientId=940&activeIngredientName=MELATONIN (accessed September 6, 2013).

12. SwansonVitamins.com, "Suzanne Somers and the 5 Supplements You Need," March 10, 2009, http://swansonvitamins.blogs.com/swanson_weblog/2009/03/i-dont-remember-a-day-like-this-since-i-began-working-for-swanson-health-products-back-in-1996-the-weather-is-so-bad-here-in.html (accessed September 6, 2013).

13. American Cancer Society, "Colorectal Cancer Early Detection," Cancer.org, http://www.cancer.org/cancer/colonandrectumcancer/moreinformation/colonandrectumcancerearlydetection/colorectal-cancer-early-detection-risk-factors-for-crc (accessed September 6, 2013).

14. Matt Kaeberlein, Thomas McDonaugh, Birgit Heltweg, et al., "Substrate-Specific Activation of Sirtuins by Resveratrol," *Journal of Biological Chemistry* 280, no. 17 (April 29, 2005): 17038–17045.

15. Barbara Brewitt, James Hughes, Elizabeth Welsh, and Robert Jackson, "Homeopathic Human Growth Hormone for Physiologic and Psychologic Health," *Alternative and Complementary Therapies* 5, no. 6 (December 1999).

16. On Line Pharmacy UK, "HGH Supplement Information," http://www.on-linepharmacyuk.com/hghsupplements.htm (accessed September 6, 2013).

17. GHRP2.com, "Human Growth Hormone (HGH) Replacement Therapy," http://www.ghrp2.com/human-growth-hormone.php (accessed September 6, 2013).

18. HormoneLogics.com, "HGH Education," http://hormonelogics.com/hgh/hgh-education/ (accessed September 6, 2013).

19. As related in "HGH—Antiaging Breakthrough? Or Hype?", http://www.i-care.net/hgh-benefits.html (accessed September 6, 2013).

20. GHRP2.com, "Human Growth Hormone (HGH) Replacement Therapy."

21. Anna Azvolinsky, "Could a Drug Prevent Brain Aging?", LiveScience.com, May 21, 2013, http://www.livescience.com/34567-calorie-restriction-drug-brain-aging.html (accessed September 6, 2013).

22. As quoted in Brad, "How to Stimulate Growth Hormone Naturally," *Applied Movement* (blog), February 16, 2011, http://www.appliedmovement.com/node/119 (accessed August 30, 2013).

23. "6 Ways to Boost Growth Hormones," part 13, page 83, http://www.herbal-pt.com/fotoy8/imagens/11–Height_Gain_Exercises.pdf (accessed September 6, 2013).

24. SelfGrowth.com, "Six Proven Ways to Boost Human Growth Hormone Output Naturally!", http://www.selfgrowth.com/articles/Staff1.html (accessed September 6, 2013).

25. Ikram Abidi, "Mastering the 'Master Hormone,'" 48, http://www.boosthgh.com/members/boosthgh.pdf (accessed September 6, 2013).

26. K. Kasai, H. Suzuki, T. Nakamura, H. Shiina, and S. I. Shimoda, "Glycine Stimulated Growth Hormone Release in Men," *ACTA Endocrinologica (Copenhagen)* 93, no. 3 (March 1980): 283–286.

27. "6 Ways to Boost Growth Hormones," part 13, page 84.

28. SelfGrowth.com, "Six Proven Ways to Boost Human Growth Hormone Output Naturally!"

Chapter 8
As a Man Thinks...

1. BrainyQuote.com, http://www.brainyquote.com/quotes/quotes/t/thomasjeff120994.html (accessed August 30, 2013).

2. Charles Kenny, "Sweet Bird of Youth! The Case for Optimism," *Time*, March 17, 2011, http://www.time.com/time/specials/packages/article/0,28804,2059521_2059564_2059561,00.html (accessed August 30, 2013).

3. Marelisa Fabrega, "Five Powerful Ways to Forgive Those Who Have Wronged You," *Daring to Live Fully* (blog), http://daringtolivefully.com/how-to-forgive (accessed August 30, 2013).

4. Masaru Emoto, *The Hidden Messages in Water* (Hillsboro, OR: Beyond Words Publishing, 2004).

5. Consumer's Research Council of America, "Prostate Cancer," http://www.consumersresearchcncl.org/Healthcare/Oncologists/oncol_chapters_2.html (accessed September 6, 2013).

6. T. S. Sathyanarayana Rao, M. R. Asha, B. N. Ramesh, and K. S. Jagannatha Rao, "Understanding Nutrition, Depression, and Mental Illnesses," *Indian Journal of Psychiatry* 50, no. 2 (April–June 2008): 77–82.

Chapter 9
Supercharged and Stress Free

1. Philippians 4:6, NLT.

2. Globe Newswire, "Workplace Stress on the Rise With 83% of Americans Frazzled by Something at Work," press release, April 9, 2013, http://globenewswire.com/news-release/2013/04/09/536945/

10027728/en/Workplace-Stress-on-the-Rise-With-83-of-Americans
-Frazzled-by-Something-at-Work.html (accessed August 30, 2013).

3. Sharon Jayson, "Who's Feeling Stressed? Young Adults, New Survey Shows," *USA Today*, February 7, 2013, http://www .usatoday.com/story/news/nation/2013/02/06/stress-psychology -millennials-depression/1878295/ (accessed August 30, 2013).

4. John Carpi, "Stress: It's Worse Than You Think," *Psychology Today*, January 1, 1997, last reviewed November 22, 2010, http://www .psychologytoday.com/articles/199601/stress-its-worse-you-think (accessed August 30, 2013).

5. Correspondence: "Mortality From Leukemia in Workers Exposed to Electrical and Magnetic Fields," *New England Journal of Medicine* 307, no. 4 (July 22, 1982): 249.

6. A. Ahlbom, E. N. Albert, A. C. Fraser-Smith, et al., *Biological Effects of Power Line Fields*, New York State Power Lines Project, Scientific Advisory Panel Final Report, July 1, 1987, http:// pbadupws.nrc.gov/docs/ML0735/ML073510363.pdf (accessed September 6, 2013).

7. Nancy Wertheimer and Ed Leeper, "Electrical Wiring Configurations and Childhood Cancer," *American Journal of Epidemiology* 109, no. 3 (March 1979): 273–284.

8. Leeka Kheifets and Riti Shimkhada, "Childhood Leukemia and EMF: Review of the Epidemiologic Evidence," *Bioelectromagnetics* Suppl. 7 (2005): S51–59.

9. Motorola.com, *Motorola Digital Wireless Guide*, www.motorola .com/mdirect/manuals/braille/V66iBraille_9464a09o.rtf (accessed August 30, 2013).

10. Ibid.

11. Ibid.

12. Nokia 6560 User's Guide, copyright © 2003, http://nds2.nokia .com/files/support/nam/phones/guides/6560_US_en.PDF (accessed August 30, 2013).

13. US Food and Drug Administration, "Radiation-Emitting Products: Interference With Pacemakers and Other Medical Devices," January 17, 2013, http://www.fda.gov/Radiation-EmittingProducts/

RadiationEmittingProductsandProcedures/HomeBusinessand
Entertainment/CellPhones/ucm116311.htm (accessed August 30,
2013).

14. Nokia 6560 User's Guide.

15. Yaniv Hamzany, Raphael Feinmesser, Thomas Shpitzer, et. al., "Is
Human Saliva an Indicator of the Adverse Health Effects of Using
Mobile Phones?", *Antioxidants and Redox Signaling* 18, no. 6 (January 16, 2013): 622–627.

16. Christopher Kent, "Models of Vertebral Subluxation: A Review,"
Journal of Vertebral Subluxation Research 1, no. 1 (1996), 1–6,
as compiled and viewed at http://www.chiro.org/LINKS/FULL/
Models_of_Vertebral_Subluxation.shtml (accessed September 6,
2013).

17. Cascade Wellness Clinic, "Benefits of Chiropractic," http://www
.cascadewellnessclinic.com/benefits.shtml (accessed September 6,
2013).

18. Sam Murphy, "Why Barefoot Is Best for Children," *The Guardian*,
August 9, 2010, http://www.guardian.co.uk/lifeandstyle/2010/
aug/09/barefoot-best-for-children (accessed August 30, 2013).

19. About.com, "Sports Medicine," http://sportsmedicine.about.com/
od/runningworkouts/a/Barefoot-Running.htm (accessed September
6, 2013).

Chapter 10
Super Natural Power to Live a Whole and Healthy Life

1. BrainyQuote.com, http://www.brainyquote.com/quotes/quotes/w/
williamart110017.html (accessed August 30, 2013).

2. "The Feynman Double Slit," http://www.upscale.utoronto.ca/
GeneralInterest/Harrison/DoubleSlit/DoubleSlit.html (accessed
September 6, 2013).

3. The Physics Classroom, "Light Absorption, Reflection, and Transmission," http://www.physicsclassroom.com/class/light/u12l2c.cfm
(accessed September 6, 2013).

Chapter 11
Twenty-One Days to Super Natural Health

1. ThinkExist.com, "Abraham Lincoln Quotes," http://thinkexist
   .com/quotation/surely_god_would_not_have_created_such_a_
   being_as/12576.html (accessed August 30, 2013).

2. Josh Clark, "Which Country's People Have the Longest Life Expectancy and Why," HowStuffWorks.com, http://science
   .howstuffworks.com/life/human-biology/life-expectancy.htm (September 19, 2013).

3. Edmond Bordeaux Szekely, *The Essene Science of Fasting* (n.p.:
   International BiogenicSociety, 1990), http://www.essene.com/
   GospelOfPeace/fasting.html (accessed September 19, 2013).

4. Bastyr University, "Feeding the Spirit: Nutritionist Helps Tribes
   Rediscover Traditional Foods," February 9, 2012, http://www
   .bastyr.edu/news/general-news-home-page/2012/02/feeding-spirit
   -nutritionist-helps-tribes-rediscover-traditional (accessed October
   16, 2013).

Chapter 12
Twenty-One-Day Jump Start Meal Plan and Recipes

1. Adapted from Nash's Organic Produce, http://nashsorganicproduce
   .com/recipes/corn-salsa/ (accessed October 30, 2013).

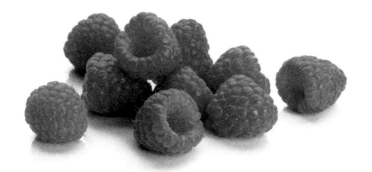

A Healthy Life—
body, mind, and spirit—
IS PART OF GOD'S PURPOSE FOR YOU!

Siloam brings you books, e-books, and other media from trusted authors on today's most important health topics. Check out the following links for more books from specialists such as *New York Times* best-selling author Dr. Don Colbert and get on the road to great health.

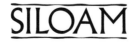

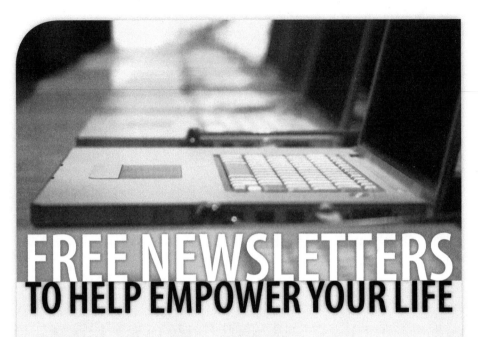